BREAST CANCER ANSWERS

Understanding and Fighting Breast Cancer

Bruce A. Feinberg, D.O.

PRESIDENT/CHIEF EXECUTIVE OFFICER
GEORGIA CANCER SPECIALISTS

JONES AND BARTLETT PUBLISHERS

Sudbury, Massachusetts

BOSTON   TORONTO   LONDON   SINGAPORE

World Headquarters

Jones and Bartlett Publishers
40 Tall Pine Drive
Sudbury, MA 01776
978-443-5000
info@jbpub.com
www.jbpub.com

Jones and Bartlett Publishers
Canada
2406 Nikanna Road
Mississauga, ON L5C 2W6
CANADA

Jones and Bartlett Publishers
International
Barb House, Barb Mews
London W6 7PA
UK

The authors, editor, and publisher have made every effort to provide
accurate information. However, they are not responsible for errors,
omissions, or for any outcomes related to the use of the contents of
this book and take no responsibility for the use of the products described. Treatments and side effects described in this book may not be
applicable to all patients; likewise, some patients may require a dose or
experience a side effect that is not described herein. The reader should
confer with his or her own physician regarding specific treatments and
side effects. Drugs and medical devices are discussed that may have
limited availability controlled by the Food and Drug Administration
(FDA) for use only in a research study or clinical trial. The drug information presented has been derived from reference sources, recently
published data, and pharmaceutical research data. Research, clinical
practice, and government regulations often change the accepted standard in this field. When consideration is being given to use of any drug
in the clinical setting, the healthcare provider or reader is responsible
for determining FDA status of the drug, reading the package insert, re-
viewing prescribing information for the most up-to-date recommendations on dose, precautions, and contraindications, and determining the
appropriate usage for the product. This is especially important in the
case of drugs that are new or seldom used.

Library of Congress Cataloging-in-Publication Data

Feinberg, Bruce A.
  Breast cancer answers / Bruce A. Feinberg.
     p. cm.
  ISBN 0-7637-3465-9
  1. Breast--Cancer--Popular works. I. Title.
  RC280.B8F44 2005
  616.99'449--dc22

                                        2004024970

Production Credits

Executive Editor: Chris Davis
Production Director: Amy Rose
Associate Production Editor: Renée Sekerak
Editorial Assistant: Kathy Richardson
Marketing Manager: Matthew Payne
Manufacturing Buyer: Therese Bräuer
Interior Illustrations: Bernie Kida and Imagineering
Composition: Lenz, Decatur, Georgia
Original Cover Design: Scott Sanders
Photo Research: Kimberly Potvin
Printing and Binding: Courier Kendalville
Cover Printing: Courier Kendalville

Printed in the United States of America
09 08 07 06 05   10 9 8 7 6 5 4 3 2 1

To Iris, Jon, Michael, Rachel, and Daniel,
Whose honesty keeps me humble;
Whose humor makes me laugh;
Whose love sustains me.

TABLE OF CONTENTS

TABLE OF CONTENTS (continued)

Preface

I am a MEDICAL ONCOLOGIST, a doctor who specializes in the TREATMENT of CANCER. After more than 20 years of patient care, I remain amazed by how little most people know about how their bodies work. Despite access to information via books, television, and the Internet, most people know much more about how their cars and appliances work than they do about their bodies. Even more surprising are people's responses when their bodies are broken. Most people will not hesitate to get two opinions about a funny noise in their car engine before forking over $1,000 to fix it. Ironically, these same people will go to the first doctor to whom they are referred and undergo a $10,000 potentially life-threatening procedure with no questions asked.

The car is a mechanical machine, whereas the body is an organic machine, albeit more complex, but not impossible to understand. I have observed that my patients who understand how their bodies normally work and how they are affected by disease feel more in control when they face serious illness. No disease is more serious than cancer, and none makes a patient feel less in control. My hope is that this book provides patients, their families, and their caregivers with the information that they need to gain control and to participate in critical decision making. Hopefully, as an active participant in their care, patients can improve their outcomes.

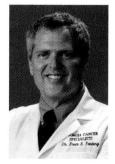

Dr. Bruce A. Feinberg

Acknowledgments

This book would not be possible without the guidance, support, knowledge, wisdom, and friendship of Richard Lenz. Richard, more than anyone, helped me translate the passion with which I educate my patients into a vehicle with which to educate breast cancer patients everywhere.

I am indebted to Melissa Faye Greene, whose validation of my work helped me persevere when I was at my lowest; Linda Loewenthal, who helped me understand the need to humanize science; and Estee Kunis, whose unqualified support gave me strength and confidence.

I thank Bernie Kida, who created the remarkable illustrations for chapter one and helped set the narrative tone of the book. I would be remiss not to mention Chris Lybeer, a cancer survivor, friend, and constant resource who, among his many contributions, introduced me to Bernie. My appreciation is also extended to Jack Haley and his team of illustrators at Imagineering, who were able to capture Bernie's tone and complete the illustration content of the book.

To Jan Galleshaw, my friend and colleague: you are the epitome of the breast cancer physician. I would not have considered this book publishable without your review of the scientific content; thank you. To Chris Murphy, the best breast radiologist in Atlanta and a treasured community resource: my thanks for helping assemble the mammograms. To my physician colleagues at Georgia Cancer Specialists: your compassionate and knowledgeable patient care is a continuous source of pride that has helped me grow as both a physician and a human being.

To Chris Davis, who took a chance on a private practice physician with a short resume: I am humbled by your confidence, inspired by your vision, and grateful to be under your wing. To the staff of Jones and Bartlett Publishers: thank you for making this book a reality. To John, Scott, Michael, Pam, Ryan, and the rest of the foosball crew at Lenz Marketing: thank you for helping to create the comp that brought my vision to life.

Finally, I need to express my gratitude to the many patients who have entrusted their cancer care and their lives to my team of caregivers. I continue to be inspired by your courage and humbled by your grace. Physicians too often forget the gifts of knowledge and skill that allow them to help others during their time of need. I remember these gifts every day.

How To Use This Book

Breast Cancer Answers is an outgrowth of my consultations with newly diagnosed breast cancer patients. Over the years it has become clear to me that simple illustrations were very effective in clarifying and reinforcing the explanations that I offered patients. My efforts to explain how the cancer began, how fast it was growing, whether had it spread, etc., were specifically enhanced with the illustrations. Despite the juvenile quality of my art, my patients often requested copies of the pencil drawings, as they helped them explain their situation to family and friends. One of my nurses suggested that I videotape a new patient discussion to improve my efficiency in the office, but I dismissed the notion as it seemed too impersonal. The suggestion did, however, trigger the thought that it would be wonderful if such a video or book were available for patients and families to have as a resource before and/or after the initial oncologic evaluation. I searched bookstores and web book retailers but could not find such a book. There seemed to be a real need for a breast cancer primer for patients. Breast Cancer Answers is designed to be such a primer. Each chapter builds on the information from the prior chapter. Illustrations accompany the narrative to reinforce and clarify the content. Keywords are in red, indicating that they can be found in the glossary for future reference.

My favorite book in medical school was an anatomy text that was illustrated with layered transparencies. With the pages in place, the image was of a human body. When the first transparency was lifted, the skin was peeled away, exposing the underlying musculature. When the second transparency was lifted, the muscles were gone, and the skeleton was exposed. Subsequent transparencies exposed the ORGANS, the circulation, and the nervous systems. My hope is that this book peels away the confusion that confronts patients and their loved ones as each layer of the breast cancer problem is revealed.

To the Newly Diagnosed Patient

Y ou have just been informed you have cancer. You are in shock. Your life is suddenly turned upside down. Don't panic! As ridiculous as it sounds, this is the best advice I can offer. To overcome the panic, you have to understand what is happening and what is going to happen to you. Your panic is rooted in the fear of the unknown and an irrational response to a situation of which you have no knowledge, no experience, and no control. Worse, you have only limited knowledge or indirect experience from cancer situations that are totally unrelated to the one that you are experiencing now. You are a newly diagnosed breast cancer patient, and your father's lung cancer and Aunt Ethel's leukemia are as different in behavior and outcome as are ice cream and artichokes.

In order not to panic and to gain control, you need to be educated about what has happened to your body and what should be anticipated. Unfortunately, seeking knowledge from well-intentioned friends and family or via the Internet is more likely to confuse than to comfort. Do not panic! With this book, the knowledge that you need to approach this disease with a positive attitude is provided.

Many types of cancer exist. With all cancers, cells in the body change and grow out of control. Usually, the multiplying cancer cells form a lump called a cancerous TUMOR. Cancerous tumors are also called malignant tumors. Sometimes MALIGNANT tumor cells can break away from the mass and travel through the bloodstream or LYMPHATIC SYSTEM to other parts of the body. This process is called METASTASIS. Not all tumors are cancerous. Those that are not are called BENIGN. Cells from benign tumors do not spread to other parts of the body.

These statements seem straightforward enough and are probably adequate for the majority of people who have not encountered the most dreaded three words in the human language: You have cancer! However, when I am in the unfortunate situation of having to say these words to a new patient and his or her anxious loved ones, this explanation is woefully inadequate. Those involved need to know so much more. The questions are endless: Where did it come from? Why did it happen to me? When did it start? How far has it gone? How big is it? Has it spread? How can it be stopped, treated, and cured? For those who are actively battling breast cancer or who are supporting a spouse, child, parent, loved one, or friend who is suffering with breast cancer, this book is for you. This is the what, where, when, why, and how of breast cancer that hopefully will make sense of everything that you have heard, seen, been through, or are about to experience. In short, I hope to answer all of the questions about breast cancer that you may have—hence the title, *Breast Cancer Answers*.

Cancer is the most complex of human diseases. It begins with a step-by-step transformation of a single human cell. Because there are over 200 types of cells in the human body, over 200 types of cancer exist, each one distinct. How can we begin to understand the more than 200 most complex human diseases? First, we turn our attention to just one cancer, breast cancer. Then, we begin as the cancer does, with a single cell. We begin by examining the origin of a human cell and the progression to the 200 different types of cells that make up a complete body. We learn about the cells that make up the breast and their normal structure and function. We examine how their behavior changes as they transform into a cancerous or malignant state. We discuss what causes this transformation as we explore cellular DNA, the genetic blueprint, or operating code that governs the cell's behavior. We describe the natural history of breast cancer and how we use this knowledge to predict a cancer's course and plan its THERAPY. We present the current strategies that medical science uses to both treat and prevent cancer. Finally, we try to make sense of the gobbly gook of jargon, terms, and statistics that can either paralyze patients with fear or confuse them with false expectations.

Read this book cover to cover. Do not skip. Do not browse. Do not wander. I have specifically written this book to provide a step-by-step understanding of breast cancer. Like the layered transparencies of my college anatomy text that peeled away the external structure to reveal the inner workings, this book explains the transformation from the normal breast to breast cancer with all of its implications. The narrative is accompanied by illustrations that will assist you as you journey through the complicated world of medical jargon and statistics. Important key words and terms are in red and can be found in the glossary. Take pauses to digest each chapter; read, go back, and reread if needed, but read methodically chapter by chapter. Use the illustrations found in each chapter to clarify and reinforce the narrative. This book is designed to be read in one evening and is going to eliminate hours, days, and weeks of emotional agony. Don't panic! Read this book!

SECTION 1

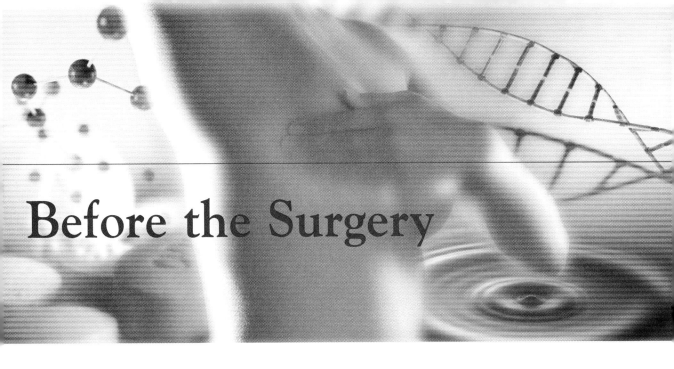

Before the Surgery

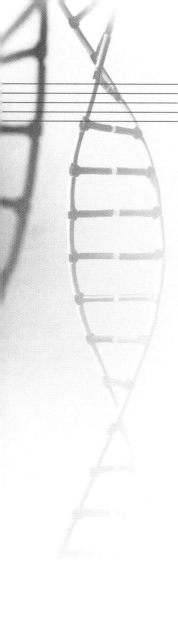

Introduction

Medical oncologists are physicians who take care of cancer patients. Most medical oncologists, like me, restrict their practice to adult cancer patients. The most common cancers are those that originate in the body's organs, such as the breast, colon, prostate, and lung. Rarely a week goes by that I do not see a new patient with a recently diagnosed breast cancer. Jill was such a patient.

Jill is 37 years old. She is the mother of Josh and Amy, ages 7 and 9 years, and wife to Greg for 10 years. Life has been good. Jill worked as a lawyer until Josh was born and recently returned to work part-time for a community agency. Eight weeks ago, Jill had her annual routine physical and pap smear with her gynecologist, Dr. Scott. Almost as an afterthought, Dr. Scott suggested that she might consider getting a baseline MAMMOGRAM. He does not normally recommend a baseline mammogram until his patients are 40 years old, which is considered the standard of care unless the patient has had an abnormal exam or a family history of breast cancer; Jill had neither. Maybe a remote patient experience or an article that he had recently read in one of his medical journals triggered the suggestion. He assured Jill that he was not hiding anything from her; her breast exam was very unremarkable. "We'll get a baseline now and then at age 40 begin annual surveillance," he said. It all seemed so innocent and matter of fact.

Jill scheduled the mammogram to be done in five weeks when there was a convenient opening at the Women's Health Imaging Center. Jill had little trepidation; it was, after all, routine, like her annual pap smear. The mammogram was a bit uncomfortable, and although the procedure took only a few minutes, getting to and from the imaging center, checking in, and waiting to be examined consumed half of the day. By the time Josh and Amy got home from school, the experience was forgotten. She was told that a nurse from Dr.

Scott's office would call in a few weeks to tell her that the mammogram was okay, as the office nurse does after her annual pap smear.

Dr. Scott himself called the next day. Jill's apprehension began with the sound of his voice, and panic erupted as he explained that there was an abnormality on the mammogram. He wanted her to go back to the imaging center that afternoon for some additional mammograms and an ULTRASOUND. She put down the phone, called Greg, and started to cry. They met at the imaging center. After the tests, a radiologist began to explain the findings. The radiologist showed Jill and Greg the mammogram abnormalities on a view box. Jill spoke to Dr. Scott, and an appointment was made to see a breast surgeon three days later. All of her fears were supposed to be assuaged by Dr. Scott's reassurances: "It's probably nothing, but we just want to be sure," and "God forbid, if it is anything, you are very lucky because it was found early." *It!* "The *it* the doctors are speaking of is cancer. What kind of luck is that? I am 37, with two small children and I have cancer," Jill thought.

In shock and silence, Jill and Greg drove home. The kids returned home from school, and Jill and Greg compartmentalized their anguish. That evening, after Josh and Amy went to sleep, Jill began making phone calls to the few friends and family who she knew had some personal experience with cancer. Doctors, hospitals, Internet sites, and alternative therapies were recommended with conviction. Jill was overwhelmed. She took a deep breath and tried to sort out what was happening. She resolved to proceed with Dr. Scott's plan but also to seek a second opinion. In the morning, she made an appointment with a second surgeon.

By the time I met Jill and Greg, three weeks had elapsed since that infamous day when the possibility of having cancer was introduced into their good life. A BIOPSY had been performed on the right breast, two surgical opinions rendered, and a reconstructive surgery evaluation scheduled. Despite the time, energy, and multiple professional opinions, Jill and Greg, an intelligent, well-educated couple, had more questions than answers. They were in my office because the second surgeon raised the possibility that Jill may be genetically predisposed to breast cancer. Before making a final decision regarding the type of breast surgery, the second surgeon suggested that genetic testing should be performed. They were completely surprised when I mentioned that chemotherapy might be needed after surgery. The questions and concerns were endless. Which surgical option was best LUMPECTOMY, MASTECTOMY, or BILATERAL MASTECTOMY? Should the reconstruction be immediate or delayed and what kind of reconstruction would be best? Would radiation therapy be necessary, and if so, would it impact the choice and timing of reconstruction? Why would she need chemotherapy after surgery? Why had the other doctors not mentioned it, and if it was needed, what kind and for how long? Was there a genetic predisposition of cancer? Why did it happen? When did it happen? How did it happen?

I have been seeing couples like Jill and Greg every week for nearly 20 years. I share their anguish; I see their pain. They had suffered through three weeks of anxiety and fear—an emotional suffering that was to continue for possibly another two to three weeks until the results of surgery would dictate final treatment recommendations. Despite family and friends, the physician consultations, books, and the Internet, patients like Jill and Greg remain in the isolation of the unknown, their minds inextricably fixating on the worst-case scenario. Jill and Greg and the tens of thousands of people like them cannot find comfort or calm their irrational fear until they understand the physical process related to this odyssey. They need the time to digest the myriad of pieces of information thrown at them, and they need the fact filtered from the fiction. They need the information accessible to digest at their pace, not in the 30 minutes allotted to them in the doctor's office. That is what this book does. This book is for every Jill and Greg, their parents and siblings, their caring friends, and their children. It is for the 250,000 newly diagnosed breast cancer patients this year and the three million women living with a diagnosis of breast cancer in the United States.

Let me explain to you the way I explained to Jill and Greg what happened to her body that resulted in a breast cancer diagnosis.

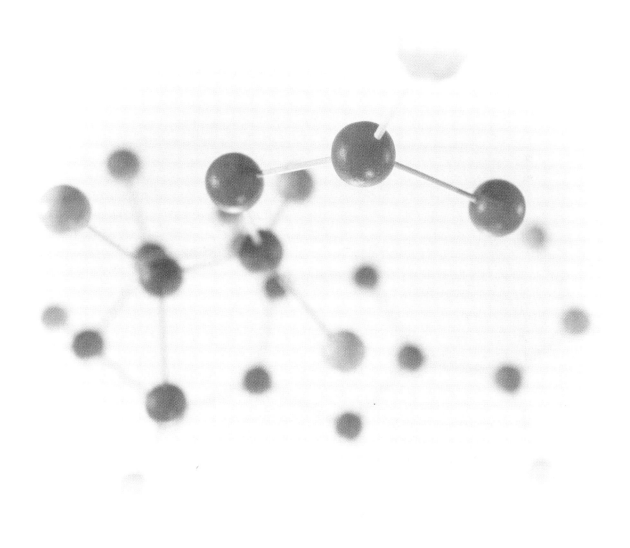

Chapter One

The Basic Science of Breast Cancer

The Cell

I have always believed that to understand what really happens to the body when it is stricken with disease you have to have some basic understanding of biology as well as human anatomy and physiology. Unfortunately, discussing such subjects can be rather dry and complicated. During such discussions my patients often echo my wife, who is fond of saying, "Just tell me the time, not how to build a clock." Even as I considered writing this book, I was still struggling to find useful metaphors and imagery to assist my patients and possible readers in grasping the biologic principles that are critical to understanding how cancers begin and grow. Divine providence seemed to intervene when my then 7-year-old son, Daniel, asked if I would speak to his second-grade class. He explained that the class was completing a study unit entitled "Jobs," and parents were encouraged to visit the class and talk about their work. After a pregnant pause, I told him I was delighted to speak, but I was not quite sure whether talking about cancer was appropriate for 7 year olds. Daniel assuaged my concerns by relating that other parents who were physicians had already presented. One child's mother explained how she kept sick people asleep while they had surgery, and another child's father talked about how he helped people to breathe better. The gauntlet was thrown: if an anesthesiologist and a pulmonologist could do it, then so could a medical oncologist. I contacted Daniel's teacher and arranged my visit. The day approached, and I was beginning to panic that there was just no way to explain cancer to 7-year-old children. To have any hope of understanding cancer and its treatment, you have to understand that animals are made from cells, that

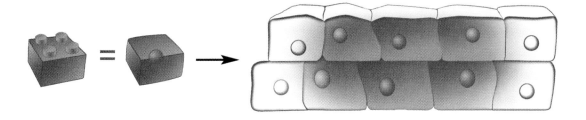

Figure 1-1: The Lego—the Perfect Metaphor for the Cell

cells can transform and grow out of control, and that medicines are available that can kill these transformed, bad-behaving cells without harming the good cells that keep us alive. Unfortunately, these kids were in second grade and did not even know what a cell was.

I went to Daniel's bedroom to confess my dilemma. Daniel was on the floor with his Legos splayed about him. When I saw the hundreds of Legos in every color, shape, and size joined in various ways to create cars, houses, and planes, I had an epiphany. The Lego was the perfect metaphor for a cell (Figure 1-1).

In Legoland, the Lego is the basic building block. Hundreds of different types of Legos when appropriately combined can create an infinite variety of structures. You can take Legos of just one variety and stack them side by side and up and down to create a wall. Add two windows and a door, and create the completed front wall of a house. After a child builds three side walls and secures them with a floor and a roof, the house takes on a recognizable appearance. Eureka, my problem was solved (Figure 1-2).

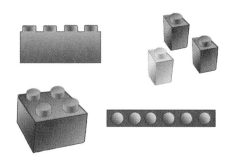

Figure 1-2: Assorted Legos

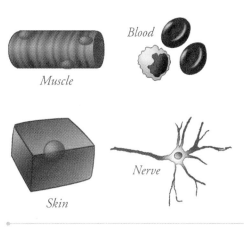

Figure 1-3: Assorted Cells

I explained to Daniel that while the Lego is the basic building block of Legoland, the cell is the basic building block of organic life (living creatures). The cell is called the origin of life because animals grow from a single cell made by the joining of sperm and egg. One cell gives rise to the billions of cells that make the complete animal. Like

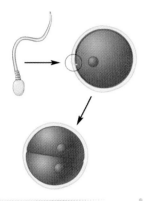

Figure 1-4:
The Origin of Life

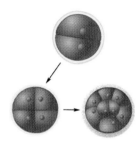

Figure 1-5:
Cellular Division

Legos, the billions of cells are not identical in appearance but rather fall into a few hundred different types: hair cells, skin cells, blood cells, etc. (Figure 1-3).

The formation of the human body, like any mammal's body, begins with the meeting of a sperm and an egg. The sperm fertilizes the egg, which creates the first cell, the beginning of a human body (Figure 1-4). This cell then divides to make two cells. Two cells divide to make four, and then those cells continue to divide until there is a cluster of cells (Figure 1-5). Initially, all of the cells in the cluster are identical. Next these identical cells begin a process in which they become the more than 200 different types of cells that make the human body complete. This process is called DIFFERENTIATION; the cells differentiate or become different types. This early developing human is called an EMBRYO.

The process of differentiation in the developing embryo begins with these clustered cells organizing into three layers: an outer layer called ECTO-DERM, an inner layer called ENDODERM, and a middle layer called MESODERM (Figure 1-6). The outer layer, ectoderm, differentiates into skin and nerve cells. The middle layer, mesoderm, differentiates into blood, muscle, and bone cells. The inner layer, endoderm, differentiates into the cells that compose all of the body's organs.

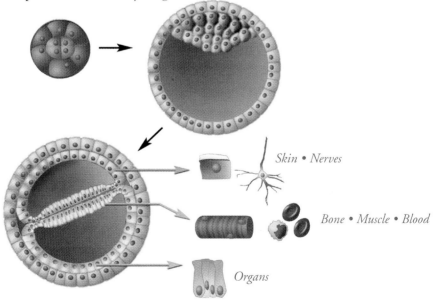

Skin • Nerves

Bone • Muscle • Blood

Organs

Figure 1-6: Cellular Differentiation

Imagine Legoland being alive. In the beginning, there was one small, rectangular, white Lego. Then there were a bunch of small, rectangular, white Legos; then white Legos morphed into three groups—purple squares and red and blue rectangles.

Primitively speaking, all of your body's organ cells begin with the endoderm layer: they have a common origin and are structurally similar. This is a very important point. As these primitive cells further differentiate and mature, their structure and function assume that of adult cells. Mature cells progress from individual cells to sheets of cells. The sheets of cells then organize to form tissues. Different types of tissues combine to form organs. Finally, the organs are arranged within a musculoskeletal framework supported by a circulatory and nervous system.

Returning to our Legoland metaphor, the white, blue, and red Legos have now morphed into hundreds of different types. There are millions of each type, billions of Legos in all. Some Legos have been assembled into a wall (like sheets of cells forming tissues). Doors and windows have been added to the wall to make the front of a house (like an organ), and roofs, floors, walls, and more have been organized to make a complete house (like a complete human being).

Daniel was an attentive and courteous listener as I expounded gleefully, progressing from Legos and cells to cancer and treatment. When I finished my diatribe, gratified to have found the long-sought metaphor, I asked Daniel what he thought. He said that he liked the Lego part but that I definitely needed to bring some kind of neat machine, like the breathing thing with the balls that go up and down. Also, I needed to bring a giveaway such as gloves or masks or maybe pencils with my name on it. I left Daniel's room defeated, feeling small and humbled. I went to my office with hopes of finding something appropriate to give 15 second graders, mired in thought of what kind of cancer machine I could demonstrate.

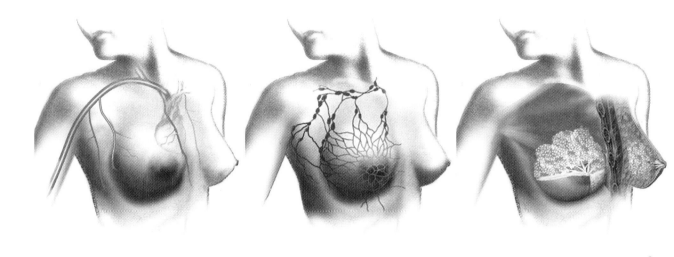

Figure 1-7 A:
Breast: Blood Supply

Figure 1-7 B:
Breast: Lymphatic Drainage

Figure 1-7 C:
Breast: Anatomy

The Breast: Normal Structure and Function

Jill and Greg were among the first patients to see my Legos demonstration, and it was a success. Not only did they not think I was crazy, but it helped them to understand cells. The next step was to explain why humans have breasts and what kinds of cells comprise them.

Unlike the Legos that I have been using for illustration, cells not only have structure, they also have function and are alive. To stay alive, cells must eat and breathe; blood provides the oxygen and food. Like the cells that comprise them, animals have to eat and breathe; they also have to reproduce or their species will become extinct. The newborns that result from reproduction must be fed before they can feed themselves. Humans are equipped with specialized cells organized into an organ that can nourish the newborn. That organ is the breast.

The breast is not an appendage like a hand or an arm. It is an organ, like a lung, liver, or kidney. You can think of an organ as having a bodily function, like the lung taking in oxygen or the kidney removing waste. The function of the breast is to produce milk for the newborn. Milk production or LACTATION requires two cellular structures: the LOBULES, which make the milk, and the DUCTS, a system of tubes that carry the milk to the nipple. The lobule cells produce the milk, which then drips into the duct so that it can flow to the nipple.

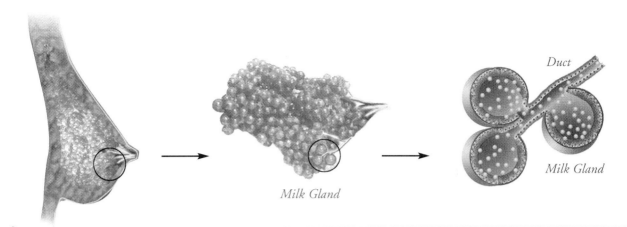

Duct

Milk Gland

Milk Gland

Figure 1-8: Mammary Tissue Magnified

The tissue in the breast that contains the lobules and the ducts is called MAMMARY tissue; a MAMMOGRAM is simply an x-ray of mammary tissue. Mammary tissue—with its blood supply and lymphatic drainage, the fibrous or connective tissue that holds it all together, the fat cells that fill the gaps, and the overlying skin—is what makes the organ called a breast (Figure 1-7). The diseases referred to as breast cancer develop in the mammary tissue within the breast. All human beings have breasts with mammary tissue, but men's breasts remain undeveloped in the absence of ESTROGENS at puberty.

Under low-power magnification, the mammary tissue is organized like bunches of grapes. Metaphorically, the grapes are the lobules that are clustered in bunches, dripping milk into their hollow stems, which are the ducts. All of the bunches and all of the stems are connected to a common vine, the nipple. A mammary duct under higher power magnification appears as a tube-like structure, a living tube (Figure 1-8). The wall of the tube is made of cells.

Throughout a woman's adult life, beginning with the start of her menstrual years, the mammary tissue is under constant stress. Month after month, the changes in a woman's HORMONE levels cause changes in the breast. These changes are physical, as well as hormonal. Before the menstrual period, the breasts become tender and swollen as the ducts dilate and the lobules enlarge in preparation for milk production if a pregnancy should occur.

Except for the interruptions of pregnancy and postpartum lactation stimulated by breastfeeding, these cyclical physical and hormonal stresses will occur for 30 to 40 years. The declining estrogen production of midlife (perimenopause) causes a regression or shrinkage of mammary tissue and an increase in the fat content of the breast. The cyclical physical and hormonal changes cease at MENOPAUSE despite the fact that a woman's body continues to produce low levels of estrogen. (Yes, postmenopausal women still make estrogen, as is discussed later.)

Jill began menstruating at the age of 13 years, nearly 25 years ago. She had never thought about her breasts as milk-making machines working continuously, albeit mostly in standby mode, for close to a quarter century. Could decades of physical and hormonal stress have caused serious problems in her mammary tissue?

Carcinogenesis

Throughout your lifetime cells are injured and repaired. Bruises, scrapes, cuts, burns, infections, chapped lips, and tongues burned by pizza cheese and hot coffee are a sample of the myriad of everyday cellular injuries that you experience. Your body has the remarkable ability to repair this cellular damage and does so in a constant, ongoing process. Some cellular damage is below the surface, caused by the tobacco smoke that we inhale, the chemicals in the food that we eat, the radiation from the sun, and the internal (natural), physical, chemical, and hormonal stresses that are part and parcel of being alive. Sometimes, if the injuries are chronic or recurrent, or if there is a genetic predisposing defect, the body is unable to repair the cellular injury. The body's failure or inability to repair cellular injury can lead to cancer. The process by which the failed repair of cellular injury leads to cancer is called carcinogenesis.

In the beginning of this chapter, I mentioned that all of the body's organs have a common origin in the cells of the endoderm of the developing embryo. As these primitive cells mature, they retain certain common features, giving organ tissue a similar appearance under the microscope. The microscopic appearance is often referred to as "glandular," which means something different than what you might think. To a PATHOLOGIST, glandular tissue is a group of cells that are organized so that they can either take in nutrients (absorb) or release chemicals needed to maintain normal body function (secrete). The cell type common to these organs is called an EPITHELIAL

CELL. The epithelial cells are flat where they connect the organs to the outside, such as at the mouth and anus; are cube shaped in the organs that are secretory, such as the breast, prostate, and pancreas; and are elongated cube shaped or column shaped in the organs that absorb nutrients, such as the colon and small intestine. When flat epithelial cells transform into cancer, they are called SQUAMOUS CELL CARCINOMA. When cuboid or columnar cells transform into cancer, they are called ADENOCARCINOMA.

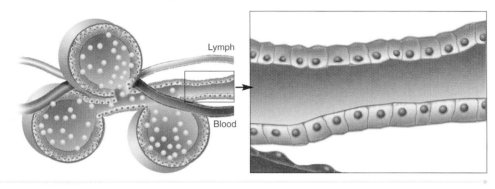

Figure 1-9: Normal Duct Cells

The glandular tissue of the breast comprised of milk glands and milk ducts is called mammary tissue; it makes or secretes milk for the newborn baby (Figure 1-9). Researchers have begun to unravel the mystery of the genetic, molecular, and cellular changes that lead to the carcinogenesis of mammary tissue. As I explain in Chapter 2, these injuries are not superficial and are not on the surface of the cell. Rather, these changes occur deep within the guts of the cell, in its nucleus and DNA, changing the cell's appearance, behavior, and very essence. They can turn a cell from its well-behaved and orderly Dr. Jekyll into Mr. Hyde, wreaking havoc and chaos. The process of transformation from Jekyll to Hyde is predictable, often slow, but always is relentless and keeps marching on.

When mammary cells transform into cancer, it is referred to as adenocarcinoma of the breast. The process begins with the hormonal and physical stress on the duct lining cells, as the ducts dilate and then contract with each normal menstrual cycle. These stresses lead to irritation and then injury of the duct cells. If the body is unable to repair the injured cells, new cells are added to the injured ones, resulting in an overgrowth of duct cells, which is called DUCTAL HYPERPLASIA (Figure 1-10).

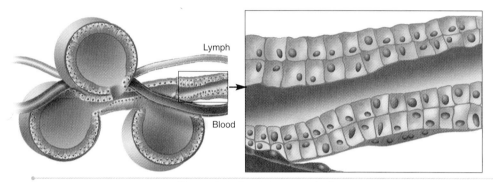

Figure 1-10: Ductal Hyperplasia

As the cells continue to overgrow, they become unstable, altering their appearance and behavior. The cells become larger and less uniform, their growth pattern less organized. At this point, pathologists call the overgrowth ATYPICAL DUCTAL HYPERPLASIA (Figure 1-11).

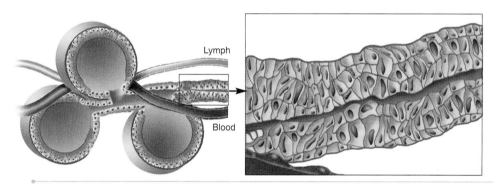

Figure 1-11: Atypical Hyperplasia

Continued stress, cellular injury, and repair process mistakes result in what are called MUTATIONS (physical changes in cellular DNA described in more detail later in this chapter), which lead to the creation of more aggressive cells. These more aggressive cells may so overgrow that they fill the entire duct space, may extend down the duct space into the lobule space, then may begin to distort and swell the duct. The packed and swollen ducts may become large enough that they can be felt on examination or seen on a mammogram. These are the characteristics of the earliest form of cancer, what is technically called DUCTAL CARCINOMA IN SITU (duct cancer within place) or DCIS (Figure 1-12). Other terms used to describe this condition are intraductal cancer and noninvasive ductal cancer.

Unfortunately, patients and doctors do not always observe distortion, lumps, or other changes on an exam or a mammogram. Not all women get mammograms, see their physician for an annual exam, or perform self-exams. Finally, neither the physical exam nor mammography is foolproof. If DCIS re-

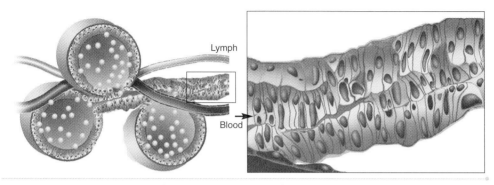

Figure 1-12: Ductal Carcinoma in Situ

mains undetected, the next event that can occur is an even more aggressive change. These unstable, mutated duct cells that have met the first criterion of cancer by their pattern of intraductal overgrowth no longer respect the boundary of the duct wall. They invade or infiltrate through the duct wall (visualize a tree root growing through the street or sidewalk). This INVASIVE DUCTAL CARCINOMA, or INFILTRATING DUCTAL CARCINOMA, is the most advanced form of cancer within the breast (Figure 1-13). (A very similar process may occur within the lobule cells leading to both LOBULAR CARCINOMA IN SITU and INVASIVE LOBULAR CANCER. However, pure lobular cancer is far less common, and the progression of lobular carcinoma in situ to invasive cancer is less clear. So we will focus on DCIS and invasive ductal cancer.)

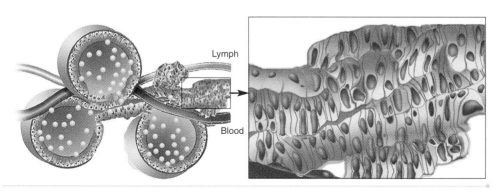

Figure 1-13: Early Invasive Ductal Carcinoma

The more I explained to Jill and Greg, the more questions they had. If hormonal and physical stress occurs in the breasts of all women, then why do all women not develop breast cancer? If these same stresses occur throughout both breasts and involve all mammary ducts, then why do only some ducts transform? I advised a deep breath and patience because I was just about to explain how physical and hormonal stress cause cellular transformation and initiate the cascade of events that result in cancer. In order to understand the how and why of carcinogenesis, one needs to understand the inner workings of a cell—its GENETIC CODE.

Genetics

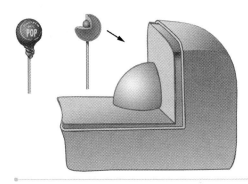

Figure 1-14: A Cell as a Lollipop

All human cells have a similar design: an outer membrane covering a gelatinous liquid cytoplasm within which is a central core structure, the nucleus. The image is that of a Tootsie Roll Pop where the wrapper is the cell membrane, the lollypop candy is the cytoplasm, and the Tootsie Roll is the nucleus (Figure 1-14). Within the nucleus resides the blueprint or operating code of not only the cell but also of the entire organism.

Like computer software written in special binary code, the operating code of living organisms is written in a special language called DNA, which is actually a chemical code comprised of four characters called NUCLEOSIDE BASES. DNA is a unique code language that, once translated, instructs the cell to build PROTEINS. Proteins are the cell's machines that bring food into the cell, remove waste from the cell, repair the cell from injury, prepare the cell for growth and division, etc.

Like many other types of machines that we are more familiar with, proteins may have many different functions but are all structurally related. Automobiles, tractors, speedboats, and helicopters are very different forms of transportation but are all propelled by an internal combustion engine. Refrigerators, blenders, washers, and coffee grinders are very different appliances, but they are all powered by an electric motor. Computers, cell phones, digital

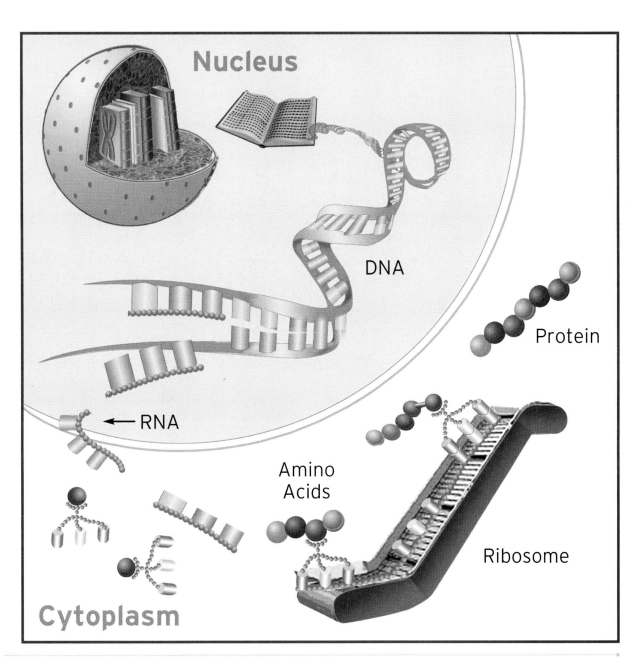

Figure 1-15: The Biochemical Basis of Life: DNA–RNA–Protein

cameras, and CD players perform different functions, but they are all controlled by a microprocessor chip. Like each of these examples of inorganic machines, proteins are the workhorses of organic machines and the cells that comprise them. The blueprint for each protein is encrypted in the DNA code.

By definition, a code must be broken or translated for the encrypted message to be understood. The DNA message for protein building requires not only translation, but it must also get transported from the nucleus to the cytoplasm where the proteins are manufactured. The translation and subsequent transport of the encrypted DNA message is facilitated by another nucleoside base language called RNA. The DNA message is translated to RNA, which leaves the nucleus and travels to the cytoplasm where it docks with a structure called a RIBOSOME, the protein-manufacturing factory.

The chemical building blocks of proteins are called AMINO ACIDS. The amino acids are chemically linked one to another according to the instructions of the DNA message. **In summary, amino acids in the cytoplasm are assembled into proteins by the ribosome under the direction of an RNA message, which is the translation of a DNA code sequence from within the nucleus (Figure 1-15).**

A complete DNA sequence that encodes a protein is called a GENE. Genes are clustered into long strands of DNA called CHROMOSOMES, which are made even longer because these genes are also separated from one another by non-message base sequences. There are 46 chromosomes in a normal human cell, 23 contributed by the father via the sperm and 23 contributed by the mother via the egg. The chromosomes are arranged in 23 pairs. Scientists now believe that there are at least 20,000 to 40,000 genes necessary for human life, making it likely that there are approximately 1,000 to 2,000 genes per chromosome pair.

Think of this genetic operating system or GENOME as the body's complete information encyclopedia. The encyclopedia is comprised of 23 volumes (chromosome pairs), each 2,000 chapters long (genes) composed in a four-character code language (DNA) requiring billions of characters (nucleoside bases) in all. Every cell in the body has the complete encyclopedia of information (genome) stored in its library (nucleus), but only certain volumes are off the shelf at any one time, opened to specific chapters as the genetic needs dictate. Genes for hair color would not be turned on in blood cells, and genes to produce insulin would not be turned on in hair cells. Beginning in the embryo and throughout cellular differentiation, maturation, and development, messages are turned on and off in a complex system of signals and responses. For the messages and signaling to work properly, every cell needs to have its billions of characters (nucleoside bases) in the correct sequence, ready for the moment when one of the volumes is taken off the shelf and opened to a chapter to be translated. A mistake in the base sequence is called a MUTATION.

Mutations can occur in a variety of ways. Sometimes information passed on from a parent is incorrect, causing some of the chapters to provide defective messages. Such genetic mutations are called HEREDITARY MUTATIONS. Sometimes there is a misprint at the factory (embryo or fetus), leading to incorrect information in some of the chapters. Such genetic mutations are called CONGENITAL MUTATIONS. Most commonly, the original information and printing are correct, but from years of use and handling, print becomes smudged, paper stained, or pages torn, leading to incorrect messages. Such genetic mutations are called ACQUIRED MUTATIONS.

Genetic defects or mutations that cause a cell to reproduce uncontrollably and invade surrounding structures are what cause cancer. Many forms of cellular injury like those caused by chemicals and radiation lead to the types of mutations that cause carcinogenesis. Mutations rarely occur from a single insult but rather from repeated insult and injury like years of tobacco use, chronic irritation, decades of cyclic hormonal stress, or just living. Thus, all cancers are consequences of genetic mutations, but few, approximately 10%, are hereditary. Most cancers are the result of acquired genetic mutations.

Was Jill's breast cancer hereditary? Neither Jill's mother nor her sister had a history of breast cancer. She was of Ashkenazi Jewish ancestry, which she knew was a RISK factor. She also knew her age at diagnosis, less than 40 years, suggested that her risk of hereditary breast cancer was greater than 10%. This is an important piece of information as it bestows a higher probability of future breast cancers and could influence choice of surgery for someone like Jill. If you are likely to have a left breast cancer or a second right breast cancer in the future, you may choose not to keep your breasts but rather have them both removed (more discussion in Chapter 3).

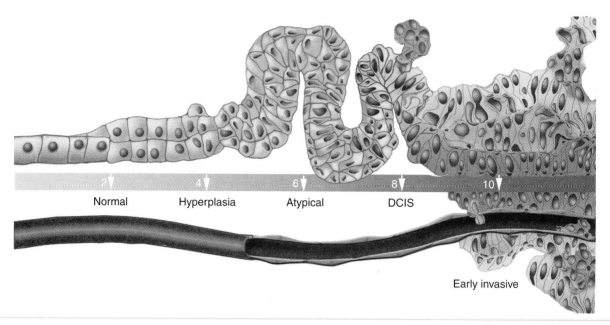

Normal	Hyperplasia	Atypical	DCIS	

Early invasive

Figure 1-16: Carcinogenesis Timeline

Breast cancer, like the majority of adult cancers, most often occurs in the sixth and seventh decades of life and is predominantly the result of acquired mutations brought about by years of cellular stress and injury. The transformation to cancer is slow, taking years or decades as gene after gene is mutated until one day the mutations are extensive enough to meet the criteria that define cancer (Figure 1-16). The most serious mutations are those that confer on a cell the behaviors of invading surrounding structures and spread through the blood and lymph circulations, as is described next.

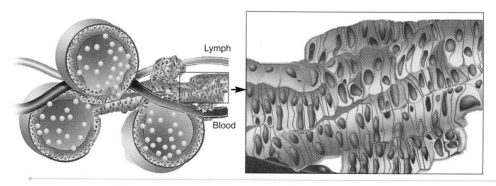

Lymph

Blood

Figure 1-17: Early Invasive Ductal Carcinoma (DCIS)

Invasion and Metastases

J
ill's normal breast exam, an absence of symptoms, and minimal mammographic abnormalities suggested that her cancer was found early, before it was invasive, at the stage of progression called DCIS. Unfortunately, the biopsy revealed a small area of invasive cancer cells (Figure 1-17). What makes invasive breast cancer more problematic is the possibility of cancer cells entering into the blood. As I explained earlier, the duct is a living tissue composed of cells. Every cell must have a blood supply to survive. Therefore, supporting the mammary tissue are blood vessels sending off small branches that nourish each of the living cells that make up the duct and the lobule.

As the invasive cancer grows through or infiltrates the wall of the duct, it may also grow through or infiltrate the wall of a nearby blood vessel. Once exposed to the bloodstream, cancer cells may break free from the growing cluster (tumor) gaining access to the blood circulation as it flows through the breast (Figure 1-18).

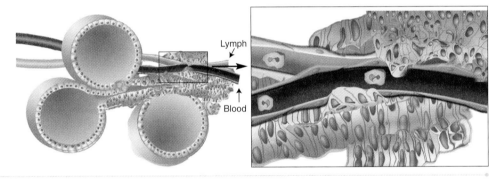

Figure 1-18: Vascular and Lymphatic Invasion

If cancer cells or cell clusters survive in the blood circulation, they may adhere to or anchor to the wall of a blood vessel anywhere in the body and there begin a new nest of growing cancer cells (Figure 1-19). This nest may then invade through the blood vessel wall (just as it originally invaded through the duct wall).

The nest may then extend through the vessel wall into the organ in which that blood vessel is located (the lung, the liver, etc.), forming a cancerous tumor in that organ (Figure 1-20). The nest of breast cancer cells anchored into a blood vessel of another organ where it then forms a cancerous tumor is what doctors call a METASTASIS (a similar process can occur within the lymph circulation of the breast, as explained in Chapter 3).

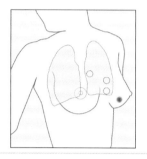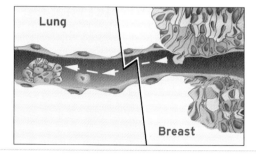

Figure 1-19: Anchored Tumor Cells

The overriding concern for the patients with infiltrating or invasive breast cancer and the doctors who treat them is whether breast cancer cells have escaped into the circulation and might develop into METASTASES. The mission of the cancer doctor is to determine the risk of metastases in order to either do something preemptively to destroy the escaping cells before they anchor, nest, and/or invade another organ (ADJUVANT THERAPY) or to treat the metastases if they can be identified or are readily apparent (METASTATIC THERAPY).

Fortunately for Jill, like most women whose cancer is diagnosed by screening mammogram, even when the cancer is invasive, cure is more likely if it is found early.

Let us return to Jill's exam, mammogram, and biopsy to understand better what occurred before she was referred and answer those nagging questions about why doctors cannot always find breast cancer during their exam, what age women should begin screening mammograms, and why biopsies are needed before surgery.

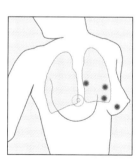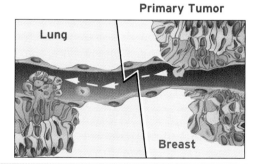

Figure 1-20: Metastases

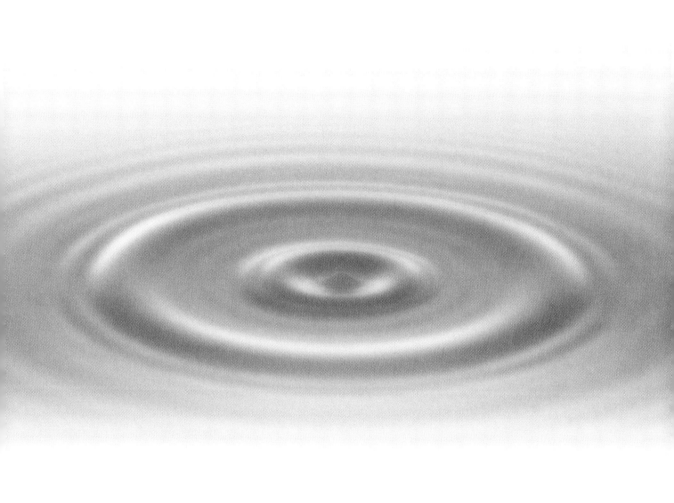

Chapter Two

Diagnosing Breast Cancer

The ultimate goal of cancer research is to prevent the disease the way vaccination has eradicated polio and smallpox. In the absence of a definitive prevention strategy, medical science's best efforts have been applied to finding or screening for the disease early enough so that it is virtually curable in 100% of those in whom it is found. Unfortunately, some cancer SCREENING tests that attempt to find the cancer early, before it produces symptoms and when it is curable, have had mixed success. Unlike the unquestioned success of the pap smear in allowing the early detection and cure of cervix cancer, colonoscopy in permitting the early detection and cure of colon cancer, and PSA (prostate specific antigen) testing in permitting the early detection and cure of prostate cancer, the screenings for breast, lung, and other cancers remain controversial.

It seems not a month goes by without a major news story about a scientific study calling into question the value of breast exams and mammograms. The elaborate and often complex scientific studies are reduced to 30-second sound bites that give the impression that women might as well just roll the dice when it comes to the early detection of breast cancer. Although I appreciate the science and recognize the need to scrutinize both the cost and value of all medical interventions, I remain steadfast in my support of early detection by the best proven means available, which today are manual breast examination and mammography.

My logic is simple. Cancer evolves from a precancerous state to a noninvasive state to an invasive state. The greater the number of cancer cells, the greater the risk of mutation to an invasive state. The greater the number of invasive cells, the greater the risk of those invading cells escaping into the circulation. The greater the number of cells in the circulation, the greater the

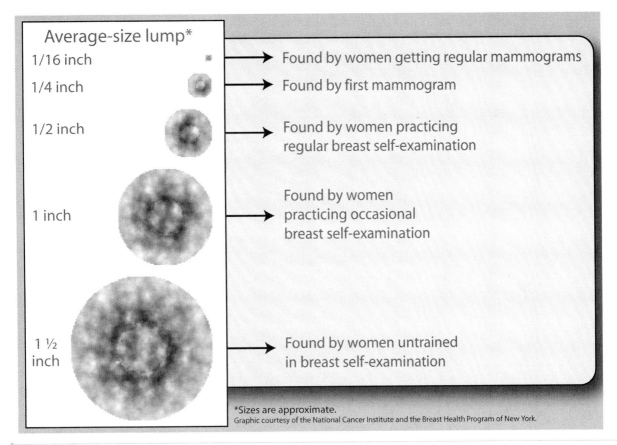

Average-size lump*

1/16 inch	→ Found by women getting regular mammograms
1/4 inch	→ Found by first mammogram
1/2 inch	→ Found by women practicing regular breast self-examination
1 inch	→ Found by women practicing occasional breast self-examination
1 ½ inch	→ Found by women untrained in breast self-examination

*Sizes are approximate.
Graphic courtesy of the National Cancer Institute and the Breast Health Program of New York.

Figure 2-1: Benefits of Regular Mammograms and Breast Examinations (The average size of tumor found with different types of screening)

likelihood that some will anchor and nest in the blood vessels of another organ, creating metastases. The greater the probability of metastases, the lower the probability of cure.

Following this logic, the key to success in cancer management is to find cancer before it is invasive, or if invasive, as soon as possible before it METASTA-SIZES. Breast self-exams, physician breast exams, and mammography are intended to do just that. There seems to be little downside to knowing your body through self-exam, undergoing an annual physical with breast exam, and undergoing age-appropriate mammography. Dr. Scott had exactly the same thoughts when he ordered the mammogram for Jill. I could say much more, but this is truly an example where a picture is worth a thousand words (Figure 2-1).

The controversy surrounding breast cancer screening relates to the concept that a screening tool must be both sensitive and specific. Numerous observations challenge the SPECIFICITY and SENSITIVITY of breast cancer screenings in younger women. First, the density of the breast tissue of a young woman such as Jill decreases the sensitivity of both the mammogram and the exam. Also, exams in young, menstruating women are notoriously unreliable because so many of the changes in the breast are not specific to cancer. Finally, the chance of breast cancer in a 40-year-old woman is very low, just 1 in 1,000, leading to a very low index of suspicion. Combined, these issues lead to problems ranging from early cancers being neither visualized nor suspected to noncancerous changes creating misleading findings leading to unnecessary biopsies and anguish. Newer and better methods are needed to screen young high-risk women, as is discussed later in this chapter.

Jill's exam was normal, and her mammogram abnormalities were at best merely suspicious given the difficulties of interpreting her young, dense breasts. The repeat mammogram involved a magnification of the suspicious area, which still was questionably a cancer. Identifying this area on ultrasound left no doubt that waiting 6 months to repeat the breast imaging was not a safe alternative. A biopsy was needed to examine the mammary cells in this suspicious area of the breast. What the doctors failed to find on exam but found suspicious on imaging and worrisome on biopsy was our next discussion.

Clinical Findings

The female breast changes dramatically with age. The flow of estrogen at puberty initiates the development of the breast, specifically the mammary tissue. The ebb and flow of sex hormones during menstrual cycles cause the breast to swell cyclically and become tender. Pregnancy produces further breast enlargement, which is fostered as long as lactation is stimulated by breastfeeding. The PERIMENOPAUSAL years are accompanied by the regression of mammary tissue and its replacement by fat. All of these changes are usually uniform and symmetrical. The hallmark of clinical breast disease is asymmetry, a visible or PALPABLE defect (clinical change) in the breast. Unfortunately, cancers that produce an asymmetrical defect of the breast are often large and advanced.

Findings of breast asymmetry—whether palpable breast deformity (lump, ridge), unilateral nipple dimpling or discharge, changes in the skin of the breast, or lump in the armpit (AXILLA)—all warrant medical evaluation (Figure 2-2). A woman who examines her breasts routinely will become familiar with the normal hormone-induced changes of her menstrual cycle and more sensitive to an asymmetrical or discrete defect as described here. A physician's exam benefits from the experience of having felt and seen diseased breasts but lacks the sensitivity of the woman who examines herself regularly. Jill had been performing monthly breast self-examinations since she was 35. She was accustomed to breast enlargement and tenderness before her menses, but she had not noted anything unusual. Dr. Scott's annual exams had also been unremarkable, but there was obviously something there. Why was a woman Jill's age not undergoing annual mammograms?

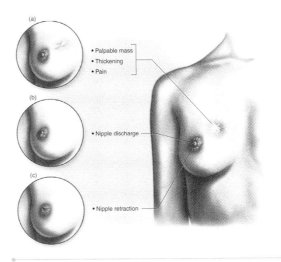

Figure 2-2: Breast Cancer: Possible Signs and Symptoms

Radiographic Findings

Radiographic testing methods were developed because asymmetry and/or a discrete clinical change of the breast may not be evident early in the development of a cancer. Scientists seeking tests that might aid in early diagnosis found that a low-dose x-ray of the breast (mammogram) may reveal distortions of the mammary tissue as well as calcium deposits technically referred to as MICROCALCIFICATIONS, which are commonly seen within regions of DCIS. Larger and coarser calcifications, discernible to a skilled mammographer, may be associated with benign breast diseases. Benign diseases of the breast, like fibrocystic disease, may be confusing to both examiner and mammographer and may require additional testing—most commonly BREAST ULTRASOUND, a technique that images the breast by sonar.

Exams and mammograms are more effective tools for detecting breast cancer in perimenopausal and postmenopausal women because in the older woman, the regression of mammary tissue and its replacement by fat increase the sensitivity of both the exam and the mammogram. The firmness or density of the mammary tissue of the premenopausal breast make the detection of a breast lump more difficult. Premenopausal breast cancer detection is further complicated by the physical changes of the breast associated with menstrual cycles. Additionally, the lower probability of cancer in the younger population makes both the doctor and the patient less suspicious. Newer techniques to image the breast, including COMPUTED TOMOGRAPHY (CT), MAGNETIC RESONANCE IMAGING (MRI), and POSITRON EMISSION TOMOGRAPHY (PET), which remain experimental as of this writing, reflect a continued com-

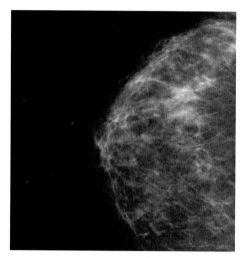

Figure 2-3 A: Normal

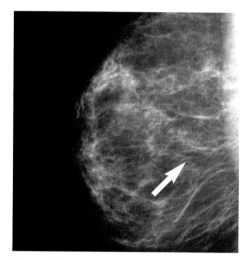

Figure 2-3 B: Micro Calcification (questionable DCIS)

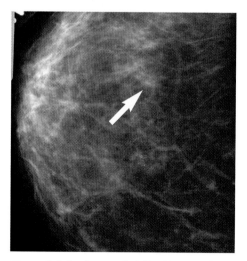

Figure 2-3 C: Coarse Calcification (Benign)

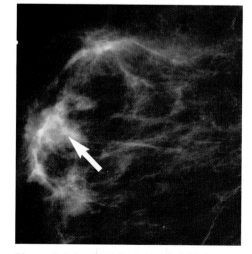

Figure 2-3 D: Stellate Lesion (questionable tumor)

mitment to improve on the early detection of breast cancer, especially in pre-menopausal women (Figure 2-3 A, B, C, D).

As I explained the limitations of breast screening in young women, Jill almost felt fortunate that the radiologist detected an abnormality. She now understood why annual mammography is not recommended until women reach the age of 40 years and why it remains controversial until women reach the age of 50 years. She also understood that for close relatives of breast cancer patients, their screening should begin 10 years younger than the age of their relative at diagnosis. This meant that her daughter Amy should undergo her first screening at age 27. That was a scary thought. I assured both Jill and Greg that in 20 years better screening tools, both genetic and radiographic, would likely be available. This seemed like a good time to discuss the genetic testing for breast cancer that is available today.

Hereditary Breast Cancer and Genetic Testing

Was there a test that could have predicted Jill's breast cancer? If Jill underwent the testing now and it proved that she was predisposed to breast cancer, would it change her choice of treatment? If Jill tested positive, should she test Amy?

If genetic events govern a cell's behavior, then genetic changes must be present before a cell transforms. However, scientists are still working to understand what changes occur among the thousands of genes in each cell that lead that cell to cancer. If a cell has 40,000 genes and just 1% of those genes mutated to confer on that cell a cancerous behavior, then 400 mutated genes would be present. If only 40 gene mutations could lead to cancer, then you would have to find 40 abnormal genes among 40,000 normal ones. Genetic testing for cancer is the ultimate needle in the haystack search. Amazingly, sometimes the detective work pays off.

After many years of scientists searching for the elusive breast cancer gene, the journal *Science*, in September 1994, announced the cloning of BRCA-1 (located on chromosome 17). This report linked mutations in the gene with breast and ovarian cancer in a handful of families. Later in the same month, a second breast cancer gene, BRCA-2, was identified in the long arm of chromosome 13. It is believed that BRCA-1 and BRCA-2 are responsible for most hereditary breast cancers. However, hereditary breast cancer is believed to account for only 5% to 10% of all breast cancer cases, as was discussed in Chapter 1.

One in every 200 women in the United States is thought to carry a defective BRCA-1 or BRCA-2 gene. The lifetime risk of developing breast cancer in a patient with BRCA-1 or BRCA-2 is 85% (normal lifetime risk = 12%). There is a 44% risk of developing ovarian cancer in patients who test positive for BRCA-1. The ovarian cancer risk of BRCA-2 is lower. As many as 30% of the women diagnosed with breast cancer before the age of 40 may be carriers of these mutations or other mutations yet to be identified.

Tests for both BRCA-1 and BRCA-2 are commercially available. Genetic counseling is the most important part of genetic screening, and in most major testing centers, more than 50% of patients who are counseled refuse testing.

Genetic counseling includes:

1. INFORMED CONSENT

2. Counseling regarding the risk of cancer

3. The availability of therapy for cancer

4. Referral back to the physician once testing has been complete

5. Post-test counseling

The individuals at high risk for the breast/ovarian cancer syndrome include those people who have two first-degree relatives (sibling, parent, child) with breast and/or ovarian cancer or three second- or third-degree relatives with breast and/or ovarian cancer. There is some suggestion that younger patients with breast cancer should be tested even without a significant family history because of their higher chances of carrying the BRCA-1 and BRCA-2 genes. Although this has not been conclusively proven, it does enable doctors to relax the testing criteria for the younger patient (under age 40 years) population. It is important to note that these are the risk factors for hereditary breast cancer and are more specific than general risk factors (Table 2-1).

As discussed in Chapter 1, all cancer is, in the final analysis, a genetic disease. Whether the cancer is the result of a hereditary mutation such as BRCA-1 or sequential acquired mutations, gene mutations are the root cause of cellular transformation. Changes in a woman's genome precede the transformation of a normal mammary cell to an adenocarcinoma. Changes in the proteins, the design of which are governed by those genes, also precede carcinogenesis. A new field of research has evolved to study the sequential changes of the gene and protein composition of mammary cancer cells with hopes that a predictive pattern of change will be observed. If such observations are successful, then it may be possible to diagnose women before the completion of carcinogenesis. This new field of gene and protein research is called, respectively, GENOMICS and PROTEINOMICS. The analysis of likely gene and protein predictors is called MICROARRAY TESTING. In the not too distant future, we may be able to create a cancer

- Personal history of breast cancer
- Family history of breast cancer, especially in first degree relatives
- Atypical ductal or lobular hyperplasia
- Early first menses, late menopause
- Late first pregnancy / no pregnancy
- Exogenous estrogens (external patches, pill)
- Radiation that has involved the breast
- Family member who is BRCA positive

Table 2-1: Breast Cancer Risk Factors

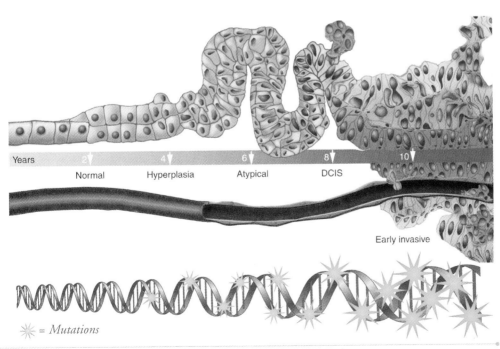

Figure 2-4: Relationship of Mutational Events to Carcinogenesis

fingerprint, a unique genetic and protein signature or bar code that identifies a cancer in development, before clinical detection and before invasion. Women found to have a high-risk gene/protein fingerprint may be treated before their cancer develops or be monitored for further mutations (Figure 2-4).

As both a daughter and the mother of a daughter, Jill decided to undergo genetic testing and counseling. Unfortunately, the testing would take two weeks to complete. Jill and Greg dreaded the thought of two more weeks of waiting. The genetic testing was important to know, as it would impact both her mother and daughter; however, would it change Jill and Greg's choice and timing of surgery? We decided to continue our discussions about her biopsy and the possible treatments that would still be needed.

Evaluation of the Breast Lump

Awoman or man with a lump or defect in the breast found on self-exam, physician exam, and/or confirmed on breast study (mammogram or ultrasound) requires prompt medical attention. Fortunately, not every lump or defect in the breast is cancer. Unfortunately, in many instances, the only way to be sure there is not cancer is to remove the defect and view the cells under a microscope. Most often, after exam and a review of the mammogram and ultrasound, the physician will perform or request a biopsy. Biopsies range from FINE-NEEDLE ASPIRATION performed in the office to surgical removal of the lump in an outpatient surgery.

When a lump is palpated or a solid defect is observed on imaging, a needle biopsy can be performed. When a fine-needle aspiration or needle biopsy is performed, the cells that comprise the defect or lump will be aspirated (sucked out) and viewed under the microscope to determine whether the cellular material is of mammary origin (not merely blood and/or fat) and whether those cells are cancerous.

Sometimes a larger needle is used to remove a slender core of breast tissue (the diameter of lead in a lead pencil). This is called a CORE BIOPSY. Specialized radiographic imaging equipment is sometimes used to facilitate the core biopsy, a procedure referred to as a STEREOTACTIC BREAST BIOPSY. Specialized biopsy devices are also employed such as a MAMMOTOME. Other times, a piece of the defect will be cut out (INCISIONAL BIOPSY) or the entire lump will be removed (EXCISIONAL BIOPSY). Regardless of the technology used, in such cases, the microscopic or pathologic review will determine whether cancer cells are present and whether they are confined to the duct space or invading through the duct wall (Figure 2-5 A, B, C, D).

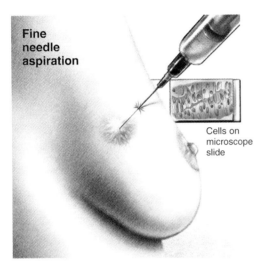

Figure 2-5 A: Fine Needle Aspiration

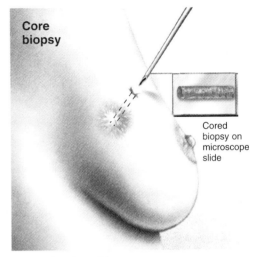

Figure 2-5 B: Core Biopsy

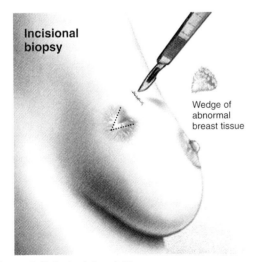

Figure 2-5 C: Incisional Biopsy

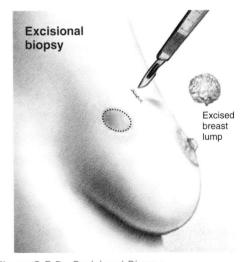

Figure 2-5 D: Excisional Biopsy

Most often, the surgeon will attempt to remove the entire defect or abnormality of the breast by performing an excisional biopsy. This is also necessary when a solid lump is not appreciated but microcalcifications are observed. The pathologic and microscopic review of an excisional biopsy must not only determine whether the cells present are cancerous and invasive but also whether all of the cancer cells have been excised. The only way to know whether all of the cancer cells are removed is to see a halo of normal cells surrounding the entire cancer lump. This halo of normal cells surrounding the diseased cells is referred to as the MARGIN. Margins will be identified as clean (uninvolved with cancer) or dirty (cancer cells extend to the edge of the specimen). A clean margin will be further categorized by the width of the halo by either measurement (e.g., 1-mm margin) or narrative (close margin). Margins are discussed in more detail later as they relate to treatment.

Regardless of the type of biopsy, this is the critical step in defining the cancer process. Cancer can be confirmed only by a pathologist's review of an appropriate specimen under a microscope. All of the x-rays and exams preceding the biopsy can only suggest or raise the suspicion of cancer. Only after a biopsy can the pronouncement "you have cancer" be made. After that, all medical efforts are directed at planning the cancer treatment. The finding of invasive cancer adds a layer of complexity to the treatment planning, as we will see in the following chapters.

Jill underwent a stereotactic biopsy, which to the surprise of the radiologist and surgeon not only revealed DCIS but also an area of invasive cancer. The cancer was not completely removed. A small piece of the tumor or core biopsy was taken to be analyzed to help Jill and Greg and the doctors select the most appropriate surgical option. Options are both a blessing and a curse, especially when they produce equal results. "Just tell me what I need to do," or "What would you do?" or "What would you recommend to your wife or mother?" are common questions. How could patients possibly decide when they feel so overwhelmed and so poorly informed? Jill and Greg had decisions to make, but first they needed to understand that surgery was not just about removing the lump of cancerous mammary tissue.

Chapter Three

Breast Cancer Treatment: History, Science, Practice

Noninvasive Versus Invasive

Unfortunately, many women's cancer is not found when it is confined to the duct, but only after there has been invasion through the duct wall. I had explained to Jill and Greg that when there is invasion there is a risk that the cancer has not only invaded through the wall of the duct but also through the wall of nearby blood vessels, thereby gaining access to the circulation and other organs. One of the greatest challenges of medical science is to develop strategies to find and destroy rogue cancer cells circulating in the bloodstream of the patient with newly diagnosed invasive breast cancer.

In many patients with invasive breast cancer, the challenge of finding rogue cancer cells in the circulation is analogous to finding a needle in a haystack. As you recall from Chapter 1, cells grow by doubling. That rogue

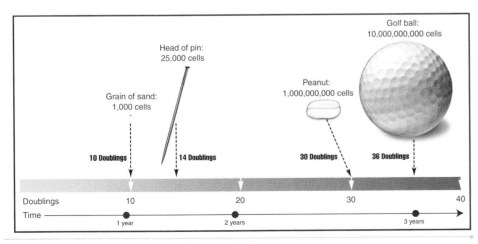

Figure 3-1: Exponential Growth of Cancer Cells

cancer cell that survives downstream will become two, these two will become four, etc. Cells are microscopic: 1,000 can fit in a grain of sand, and 25,000 can fit on the head of a pin (Figure 3-1). None of our current diagnostic studies—neither laboratory tests nor CT, MRI, and PET scans—can detect cancer at that microscopic level.

Physicians and patients are in the uncomfortable position of knowing that cancer cells may be loose in the circulation without having any proof. Any observation that might predict the probability of cancer cell contamination outside the breast is critical to planning the treatment of the breast cancer patient. The patient's age, the size of the tumor, the tumor cell's sensitivity to estrogen, and the presence of increased amounts of the gene HER-2/NEU (these features will be discussed in more depth in future chapters) have all demonstrated predictive value, but the presence of cancer cells within the LYMPH NODES of the breast is the single most important factor in predicting breast cancer cell spread outside of the breast.

Evaluation of the Lymph Nodes

Still in shock having just learned that the biopsy revealed an area of invasive cancer, Jill and Greg tried to understand as I explained the lymph system and the need to evaluate the lymph nodes under her arm.

Another type of blood channel runs alongside the blood vessels in the breast and throughout the body. These are called lymph channels. Lymph and blood are related. Blood is composed of RED BLOOD CELLS, WHITE BLOOD CELLS, and PLATELETS, suspended in a fluid called PLASMA. The red blood cells are carrying oxygen to every living cell in the body. The white blood cells are surveying for and destroying foreign invaders (bacteria, viruses, etc.). The platelets are plugging holes in traumatized blood vessels to prevent bleeding. Although all three types of cells circulate in blood vessels, only white blood cells circulate in the lymph system. If we think of the blood as nourishing all of the living cells of our body with oxygen and glucose (sugar), we might think of the lymph as washing every living cell, washing out bacteria, viruses, and anything foreign to our body that might infect or injure it. With lymph channels side by side with blood vessels, if a root or tentacle of tumor has invaded through the duct wall and through a nearby blood vessel, most likely it will invade through the lymph channel as well.

Unlike the blood, which flows uninterrupted from organ to organ delivering oxygen and nutrients to each cell it touches, the lymph is filtered between organs by structures called lymph nodes. When the white blood cells in the lymph have surrounded bacteria or viruses, these microbes are filtered out by the lymph node, where special killing cells destroy them and prevent further spread. Unfortunately, cancer cells originate (mutate) from our own cells. Despite their bizarre appearance and aggressive behavior as well as their potential to harm the body, they still appear human to the IMMUNE SYSTEM. Therefore, they are not recognized by the killing cells in the lymph node as foreign invaders, and they are not destroyed. They are, however, trapped in the node. If they are living but are trapped, they will multiply, and a nest will grow (Figure 3-2).

This is critical knowledge for doctors who are managing breast cancer patients. The lymph nodes are a window into the circulatory system and help doctors understand the potential risk for cancer spread. A pinhead-size cluster of cancer cells in a lymph node that would have escaped detection by physical examination, laboratory testing, or radiographic imaging can be found when the node is examined under a microscope. If a lymph node is contaminated by a nest of cancer cells, then the cancer invaded the lymph channel and probably also invaded the neighboring blood vessel. Lymph involvement confirms that despite removing the cancerous tumor, there may still be cancer cells contaminating the body. The greater the lymph involvement, the greater the risk.

The distinction between noninvasive and invasive ductal cancer, the predictive value of lymph node involvement, and the increasing understanding of the natural history of breast cancer has coincided with an evolution in doctors' strategies to diagnose and manage a breast compromised by cancer. Having gotten this far with Jill and Greg, the next step was to explain the different surgical options and to help them understand the differences so that they could then select the most appropriate option for Jill.

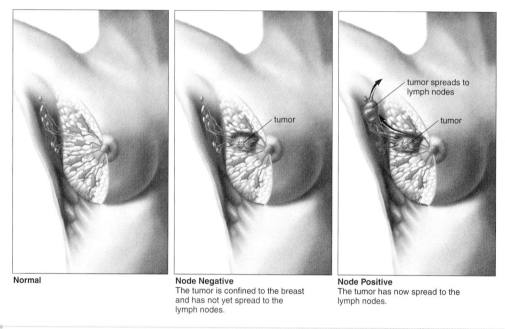

Normal

Node Negative
The tumor is confined to the breast and has not yet spread to the lymph nodes.

Node Positive
The tumor has now spread to the lymph nodes.

Figure 3-2: Breast Cancer Evolution from Benign to Nodial Spread

Evolution of Breast Cancer Management

Our understanding of cancer has changed quite a bit over the past century. It was over 100 years ago that the first effective breast cancer treatments were published. At that time, the only treatment was surgery formulated on the notion that cancer was a manifestation of a diseased organ. The only way to eradicate the disease was by radical surgery to remove the entire organ with its blood supply and lymph drainage.

The doctors of the late 19th and early 20th centuries believed that cancer would spread from the diseased organ to the draining lymph nodes and only then to other organs. Therefore, the cancer could be stopped by removing, resecting, or dissecting out all of the lymph nodes that drain the cancerous organ. The majority of the nodes that drain the breast are located under the arm in the armpit, which is anatomically called the axilla; hence, the surgery to remove all the lymph nodes from the axilla is called a COMPLETE AXILLARY NODE DISSECTION.

For nearly 100 years, breast cancer patients not only underwent complete axillary node dissection, but doctors also removed the entire breast as well as the muscles beneath the breast and the blood vessels supplying the area. This was called a RADICAL MASTECTOMY. The radical mastectomy with its requisite complete axillary node dissection was not only quite deforming but also it was associated with late COMPLICATIONS, the most serious of which was IPSI-LATERAL or same-side arm LYMPHEDEMA. Lymphedema is a swelling of the arm after its draining axillary lymph nodes have been injured by surgery and/or

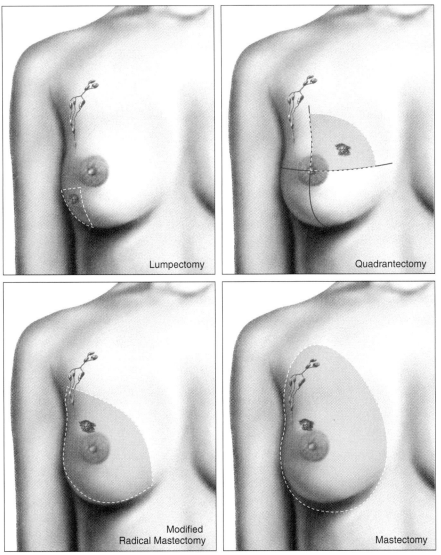

Figure 3-3:
Breast Surgery Options

Lumpectomy

Quadrantectomy

Modified
Radical Mastectomy

Mastectomy

radiation. The arm may swell three to four times normal size, causing pain and restricting motion. The lymphedematous arm is also more susceptible to infections, which is why doctors recommend that neither blood draw nor blood pressure monitoring be performed on it.

Over the past 30 to 40 years of cancer research, scientists began to realize that the cancer problem is not what you can see with the unaided eye, not merely a local or even a regional problem of an organ and its draining lymph nodes, but rather breast cancer, like all organ cancer, is a total body or SYSTEMIC disease. The cancer cells gain access to the entire circulatory system and can nest microscopically and invisibly anywhere in the body. Curing cancer was less related to the extent of breast surgery and more related to the ability of medical science to develop treatments that would destroy the breast cancer cells at large in the body.

By the last quarter of the 20th century, radical mastectomies and complete axillary lymph node dissections had become inconsistent with the new systemic theory of cancer, which stated that lymphatic involvement occurred simultaneously with cancer dissemination into the blood circulation.

Understanding the differences between invasive and noninvasive cancer as well as the emerging systemic theory of cancer helped doctors realize that they could limit the extent of breast surgery without compromising cure. Incorporating scientific theory into clinical practice led to the less deforming MODIFIED RADICAL MASTECTOMY. More recently, the desire to preserve the breast has resulted in further reductions in the extent of breast surgery, leading to BREAST-CONSERVATION SURGERY, also called PARTIAL MASTECTOMY, SEGMENTAL MASTECTOMY, and LUMPECTOMY. These organ-sparing or breast-conserving surgeries, when complemented by breast irradiation to sterilize the remaining mammary tissue, have proven equal in effectiveness to the more radical surgical approaches for nearly 90% of breast cancer patients. Preserving the breast without compromising cure has made the lumpectomy the procedure of choice for the majority of breast cancer patients (Figure 3-3).

In conjunction with reductions in breast surgery, researchers began advocating smaller lymph node samplings. They advised taking only the most likely contaminated and accessible nodes, approximately 10 on average, in a proce-

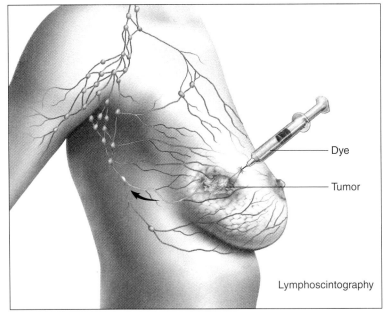
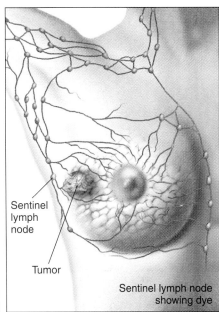

Figure 3-4: Sentinel Node Evaluation

dure called AXILLARY SAMPLING. Even more recently, doctors have recognized that lymph drainage coming from an area of the breast typically flows to one particular lymph node as the first in a chain to receive that lymph drainage. That first lymph node in the chain to receive drainage from the area of the breast lump is called the SENTINEL LYMPH NODE. Research now demonstrates that adequate lymph node evaluation can be achieved by injecting dye within the location of the breast lump (tumor), watching over 30 minutes to see which lymph node is the first to accept the dye (LYMPHOSCINTIGRAPHY), and then removing that sentinel lymph node (SENTINEL NODE BIOPSY) (Figure 3-4).

When I read or hear comments suggesting that little progress has been made in the management of breast cancer, I am quick to respond that in the past 30 years the surgical management of breast cancer has been reduced from the radical mastectomy, with complete axillary dissection, to the mere removal of a lump and a single lymph node.

Jill was clearly a candidate for breast-conservation surgery, but her eligibility was just one factor to consider in her decision-making process. Because breast conservation required radiation, she and Greg needed to know more about radiation treatment.

Role of Radiation Therapy in Locoregional Disease

Picture a pebble being tossed into a pond and the wave-like ripples that simultaneously emerge in all directions from the point of impact. Now with that picture in mind, imagine a lit candle afloat in the middle of the pond with its light radiating in all directions. Science refers to that visible light as radiant energy (Figure 3-5).

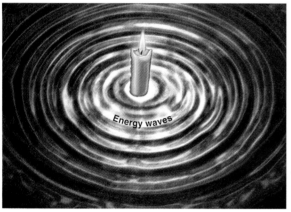

Energy waves

Figure 3-5: Radiant Energy

Like the ripples in the water after a pebble toss, radiant energy also emanates in omnidirectional waves from its source, except that these waves are invisible. Radiant energy is classified by the distance between the waves, referred to as WAVELENGTHS. Wavelengths vary, ranging from wider than a million meters to as narrow as one billionth of a meter. This mind-boggling range of radiant energy wavelengths makes up the ELECTROMAGNETIC SPECTRUM (Figure 3-6). The shortest wavelengths are those that produce therapeutic radiation. The longest wavelengths are those associated with electricity. In between

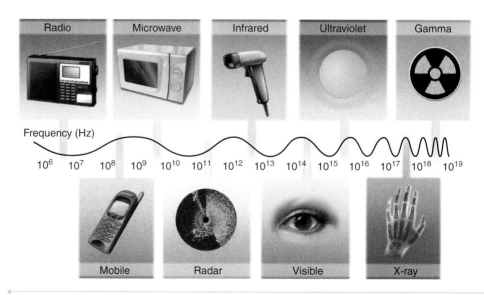

Figure 3-6: Electromagnetic Spectrum

these extremes, as we move from short to long in the electromagnetic spectrum, are diagnostic x-rays; ultraviolet light; visible light; infrared light; microwaves (radar); and television, radio, and communication frequencies.

Therapeutic radiation, also called GAMMA RADIATION, refers to the clinical use of radiant energy emitted by radioactive substances. Like the ultraviolet radiant energy from the sun that can affect skin by damaging cells on the skin surface, gamma radiation can penetrate below the skin, damaging cells internally. Computers and other equipment permit the gamma rays to be focused and contoured to a particular structure of the body like the breast. At a high enough exposure to gamma rays, cells may not only be injured but also killed. Research has revealed that when doses of gamma rays are delivered repeatedly (called FRACTIONS) to cancer cells, they will kill the cancer cells without killing the surrounding normal cells. Therapeutic radiation exploits this research to develop treatment strategies for different cancer problems.

Therapeutic radiation may play a variety of roles in the treatment of breast cancer. Most commonly, it is used to sterilize a breast of residual microscopic cancer cell contamination after a cancerous tumor has been surgically removed, thus permitting preservation of the breast (breast-conservation surgery). Even when the breast has been removed, radiation treatments may be recommended for the skin of the chest and the remaining axillary lymph nodes if the cancerous tumor was very large or if multiple lymph nodes were found to be contaminated. Finally, radiation treatments may be helpful in controlling symptoms from nests of breast cancer cells that may have grown in other parts of the body (metastases), especially in the bone.

Novel research in therapeutic radiation is now developing techniques to improve external radiation targeting, implant radioactive seeds, and inject targeted radioactive molecules. Therapeutic radiation remains a critical component of breast cancer treatment planning, as explained in future chapters.

Management of the Breast (Locoregional Therapy)

Jill and Greg had now learned about the evaluation of the breast. They understood why the lymph nodes are important and how doctors can minimize the complications from breast and lymph node surgery by using breast conservation approaches, limited lymph node sampling, and sentinel node analysis. They also understood the relationship between the extent of node involvement and the risk of metastases. Now I wanted to turn their attention to how ONCOLOGISTS integrate these treatments.

The local (breast) and regional (lymph nodes, chest wall) treatment options for breast cancer are numerous. Many factors should be considered

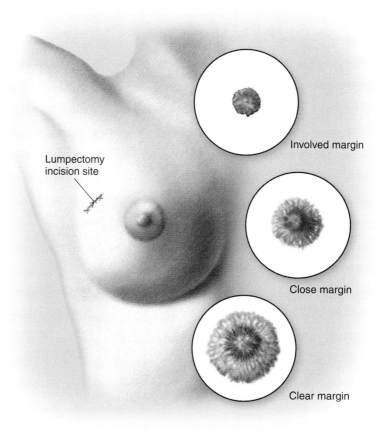

Lumpectomy
incision site

Involved margin

Close margin

Clear margin

Figure 3-7: Surgical Margins

when selecting treatment for this disease. Physician and patient preferences, patient age and anatomy, tumor characteristics (including size, location, and pathology), genetic profiling, and patient and family history are all important considerations. Although management of the involved breast and the uninvolved breast and the method of lymph node evaluation remain individually specific as is discussed later, some general comments about locoregional therapy are relevant here.

If the biopsy confirms cancer, but it is confined to the duct space (DCIS), then removing it, in theory, cures the cancer. However, removal or excision must be complete. To assure complete excision, the pathologist evaluates tissue along the edge or cut margin of the excised lump of DCIS to make sure that there is normal mammary tissue surrounding the entire focus of DCIS. If DCIS is found on any surface of the lump, it is referred to as a contaminated margin and may require further surgery to achieve complete tumor removal (Figure 3-7).

However, even when all margins are negative and the cancerous tumor has been completely removed, a problem exists: research has revealed that in other parts of the breast there could be atypical hyperplasia or even DCIS that was not yet visible on mammogram or palpable on exam. Diseased areas within other parts of the breast would then be missed if not treated at this time and could emerge later as invasive disease. Thus, not only do doctors have to remove the DCIS that was found, but they also need to treat the remaining mammary tissue in the diseased breast. The finding of DCIS in one part of the breast identifies cancer risk throughout the breast.

Currently, there are two standard ways to treat a breast with completely excised, margin-negative DCIS. One way is to remove the breast in its entirety (SIMPLE MASTECTOMY). The other way is to use high energy in the form of EXTERNAL BEAM RADIATION THERAPY to sterilize the remaining mammary tissue after the lump is completely removed by breast-conservation surgery. In patients with DCIS, doctors are not worried about spread throughout the body because as long as the cancer is confined to the duct space there is no risk of spread through blood or lymph. Therefore, lymph nodes are not removed for pathologic review.

More than 90% of patients with DCIS can choose the option of breast-conserving surgery, confident that breast preservation will not compromise the chance of cure. Mastectomy is preferred in a minority of patients: those in whom DCIS is extensive, those where DCIS location prevents a good cosmetic outcome, and those with severe fibrocystic disease which compromises future screening.

Regardless of the choice of management of the diseased breast, there remains a concern of future cancer in the uninvolved breast. Annual mammography and a physician exam as well as monthly self-exam are therefore a must. Recently, strategies have been developed to prevent new breast cancers in both the involved and uninvolved breast (discussed later in prevention). Additionally, molecular testing and genetic testing to assess risk of breast cancer are becoming available to allow those women at very high risk to choose preventative or PROPHYLACTIC bilateral mastectomy.

If the biopsy confirms that there is an invasive ductal carcinoma, as in Jill's, the situation is similar to the one I just discussed. The entire breast remains at risk and must be treated even if the tumor has been removed. Again, the option is to remove the breast in its entirety or to sterilize it with radiation, both of which has been found to be equally effective in the majority of women. However, in the patient with invasive cancer, something else still needs to be done. The lymph nodes that filter the breast's lymph circulation may hold clues to the risk that this cancer has gained access to the blood circulation. Those lymph nodes are under the arm (armpit or axilla) and need to be evaluated. Simple breast management will not be adequate here because the lymph nodes must also be evaluated. The surgical options in a patient with invasive cancer must include axillary sampling or sentinel node evaluation.

Jill and Greg clearly understood the surgical options. She was an appropriate surgical candidate for breast conservation and was not bothered by the need for radiation treatment. She could have the breast removed and undergo an immediate breast reconstruction. However, Jill and Greg remained concerned about Jill being genetically predisposed to breast cancer. Jill was seriously considering having a bilateral mastectomy followed by immediate bilateral breast reconstruction. The meeting that was scheduled with the reconstructive surgeon in the morning would help them finalize their decision.

Reconstructive Surgery

Breast reconstruction has become part and parcel to the discussion of local breast management. The breast surgeon and reconstructive surgeon work closely to optimize the surgery technically and logistically. Once a patient's general health is assessed, the reconstructive surgeon will explain which options are most appropriate based on age, anatomy, tissue, and goals. Jill was fortunate, as she had no issues in her medical history that might complicate reconstruction. She had no serious medical problems. She was not obese and she did not smoke. Jill, Greg, and the reconstructive surgeon had a frank discussion of options as well as the risks and limitations of each. She also understood the anesthesia required for each procedure.

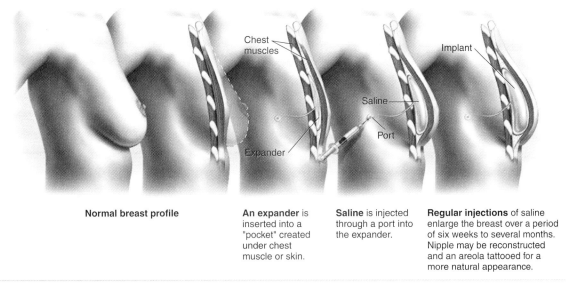

| Normal breast profile | An expander is inserted into a "pocket" created under chest muscle or skin. | Saline is injected through a port into the expander. | Regular injections of saline enlarge the breast over a period of six weeks to several months. Nipple may be reconstructed and an areola tattooed for a more natural appearance. |

Figure 3-8: Expanded Implant

Jill seemed reassured that if she chose mastectomy, the currently available techniques and devices would make it possible for the surgeon to create a breast that would come close in form and appearance to the natural breast it would replace. She also understood that reconstruction could be done immediately, during the same surgery as the mastectomy. She could wake up in the recovery room with a breast mound in place, never having the experience of seeing herself with no breast at all. She also understood that this was not a simple procedure; multiple surgeries would be needed to achieve a natural-appearing breast.

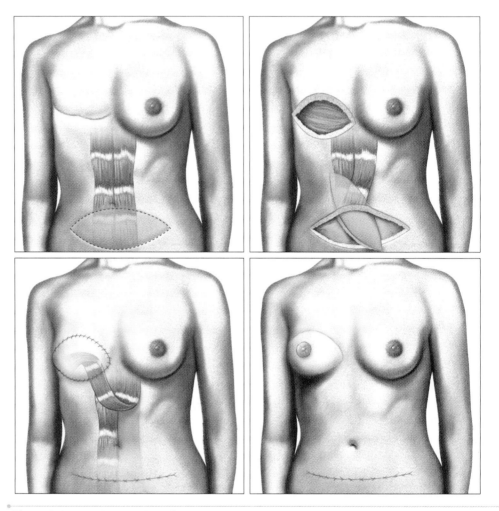

Figure 3-9: TRAM Reconstruction

Despite the obvious benefits of immediate reconstruction, Jill knew there were legitimate reasons to wait. There were so many decisions to make. Was she prepared to also make the necessary decisions regarding her reconstruction? She knew that postoperative complications of wound healing, bleeding, and infection could delay SYSTEMIC THERAPY. Even if systemic therapy was not delayed, was she prepared for the postoperative pain and the anticipated symptoms of healing?

Jill was able to summarize her options as two: an IMPLANT placed below the pectoralis muscle of the chest wall or a full-thickness transplant of abdominal skin, fat, and muscle placed over the chest wall called a TRAM flap (Transplanted Rectus Abdominal Muscle). A similar full thickness transplant of the latissimus muscle was an alternative. The implant seemed easier. A noninflated plastic bag would be inserted under the pectoralis muscle after the mastectomy and gradually filled with saline over the subsequent weeks. Once the bag held enough saline and had stretched the muscle and skin to the size of her natural breast, the saline bag would be removed and a full-size implant inserted in its place (Figure 3-8). The alternative was a transplanted flap of skin and muscle from Jill's abdomen. The full-thickness flap from her abdomen would likely cause more pain, as the abdominal wound represents a second surgery; however, it would offer a more natural feel, as only living tissue would make up her new breast. She was intrigued that a flap of skin, fat, and muscle could be removed from her abdomen but remain connected to its blood vessels and nerves as it was turned upside down to make the breast (Figure 3-9). If she chose to have both breasts removed, this was definitely the better option as far as she and Greg were concerned.

Jill and Greg were clear that regardless of the extent of surgery, her hospitalization was unlikely to be less than two or more than five days. She understood that she might go home with a surgical drain, which removes excess blood and fluid from the wound. She knew that the drain and stitches would likely be out in 10 days, but it could take six weeks before she was completely recovered. Although scars would heal and fade over time, normal sensation would never be completely restored.

Jill and Greg were satisfied. They had reached a decision. All of their questions had been answered. The following week she would undergo the following surgeries: a right simple mastectomy to remove the cancer and the involved breast, a right axillary sentinel node biopsy to evaluate for node contamination by the invasive cancer, a left simple mastectomy to prevent a future left breast cancer, and bilateral breast reconstruction with a TRAM procedure. I told her I would visit her in the hospital before her discharge to review the final pathology of the breast and nodes. I told Greg I would call him and let him know when I would stop by the hospital room so that he could be there. They were still a bit uneasy knowing that until the final pathology was reviewed we could not discuss whether or what kind of systemic therapy might be needed.

SECTION 2

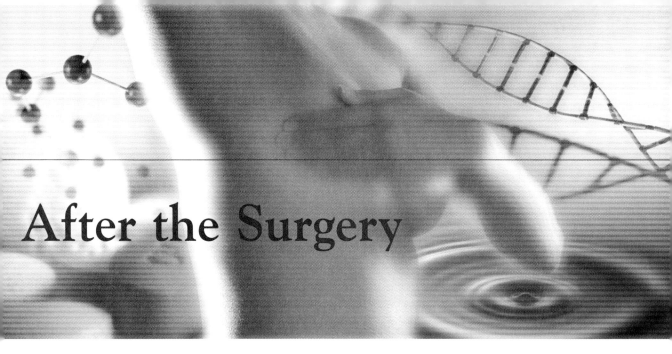

After the Surgery

Introduction

This section demystifies the postoperative return visit. We follow along with Jill and Greg as the pathology findings are organized into a quantifiable database referred to as STAGING. We review the relationship between STAGE and probability of cure. We then discuss the different types of postoperative treatments that can be used to improve the probability of cure. We review how research has improved the outcome for breast cancer patients as well as how ongoing CLINICAL TRIALS allow patients to gain access to new treatments. We try to make sense of the myriad of measurements used to assess the benefits of these systemic interventions. Finally, we offer some words of caution and common sense regarding the burgeoning field of alternative and complementary therapy. Let us return to Jill and Greg at their first postoperative visit to the office.

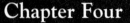

Chapter Four

Systemic Treatment Planning

Jill tolerated surgery well, without complication, leaving the hospital on the third postoperative day and before the final pathology report was available. I arranged for Jill and Greg to come by the office the following week to discuss the findings and their implication on further treatment. Unfortunately, although the breast tumor was found to be quite small, (just over one centimeter), the sentinel lymph node was contaminated. The sentinel node was found to have a small cluster of cancer within it, requiring the surgeon to sample some additional lymph nodes. Fortunately, these additional nodes were not contaminated by the cancer. As I sat down with Jill and Greg to review the final pathology reports, they asked familiar questions: Is it good or bad? Did we catch it early? The root of these questions is this: Will I be cured? Fortunately for Jill, as for the majority of breast cancer patients, the answer is yes. Unfortunately, cure does not come without a cost, as the great majority of breast cancer patients must undergo systemic therapy after their breast and lymph node surgery.

Staging and Grading

It was time for the most difficult job I have as an oncologist: to explain to the patient that although the surgeon said "he got it all," he really meant to say "he removed all of the cancer he could see;" however, microscopic cancer may still be in the body. No matter how positively I try to present the pathology findings, when the probability of cure is not 100%—and it usually is not—a cloud of gloom hangs over the discussion. Jill's chances of cure were excellent but not 100%; so, I placed a box of tissues on my desk and was emotionally prepared for our discussion.

ONCOLOGY in its essence is a discipline of medical science. In a scientific discipline, theory is tested by experiment, and success is measured quantitatively. In order to quantify the probability of cure or, inversely, the risk of cancer relapse, the oncologist must weigh the evidence that is available. The evidence may be found in the pathology reports, laboratory tests, and imaging, but it must be organized in a meaningful and comparative way. The oncologic community responded to this need by standardizing a system for quantifying cancer, both the extent of disease and the characteristics that determine the risk of relapse and the probability of cure. Although it is the physician's desire to comfort and provide hope, there is no escaping an objective review of data with a patient before they can provide an informed consent to undergo treatment.

Information gathered about the breast tumor or lump and the lymph nodes, the radiographic imaging, and the laboratory data comprise the database. The database is organized to quantify or grade (the word grade also has a technical definition that is addressed at the conclusion of the section) the amount of disease locally within the breast, regionally within the nodes, and distally within other organs. This system of cancer measurement addresses each area of disease as follows: the breast lump (tumor = T) regarding its size, extent, and location (graded 1 to 4); the lymph nodes (nodes = N) regarding number, character, and location (graded 0 to 3); and evidence of other organ spread (metastasis = M), either there is or there is not (graded 1 or 0). This is called the TNM STAGING SYSTEM.

The very least amount of invasive cancer would be represented by a very small tumor (T1), without lymph node involvement (N0), and without spread to other organs (M0), or (T1 N0 M0). The worst scenario would be any cancer that had already spread to other organs of the body (T-any, N-any, M1).

Staging allows doctors to categorize patients with similar cancer characteristics, thereby helping to predict outcomes and permitting treatment stratification based on risk. Stage I cancers are very small (less than 2 cm) and have no proven spread to lymph nodes or other sites (Figure 4-1). Cancers that are larger than 2 cm or involve regional lymph nodes are grouped into stages II and III (see Figures 4-2–4-4). Any cancer that has spread to another part of the body (e.g., lung, liver, bone) is stage IV.

NOTE: The tumor and lymph nodes represented in these illustrations are below the skin surface and may not be visible to the unaided eye.

T1 N0 M0

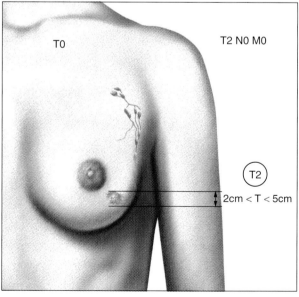

T1a: T ≤ 0.5cm

T1b: 0.5cm < T ≤ 1cm

T1c: 1cm < T < 2cm

(T1)

T ≤ 2cm

N0 + no regional lymph node metastasis

Figure 4-1: Stage I Disease

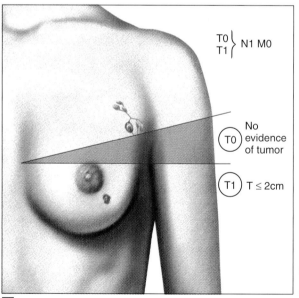

T0
T1 } N1 M0

(T0) No evidence of tumor

(T1) T ≤ 2cm

T0

T2 N0 M0

(T2) 2cm < T < 5cm

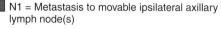

N1 = Metastasis to movable ipsilateral lymph node(s)

Figure 4-2: Stage II A Disease

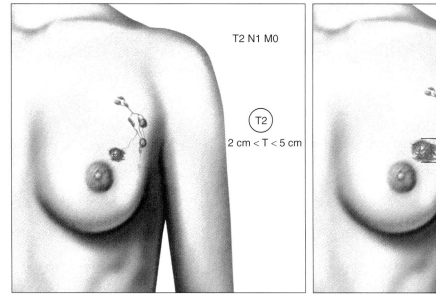

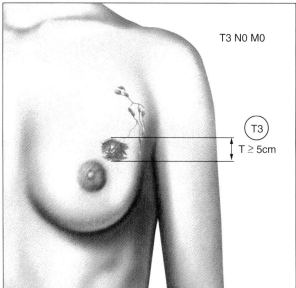

N1 = Metastasis to movable ipsilateral axillary lymph node(s)
(p) n1a, Nb

Figure 4-3: Stage II B Disease

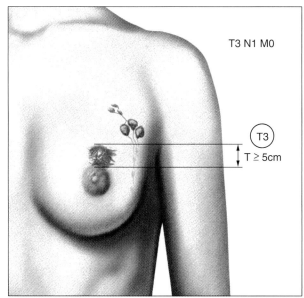

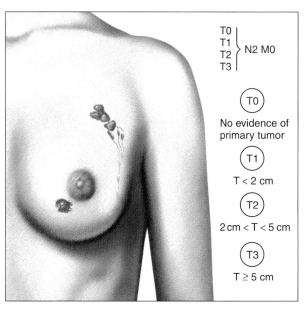

Metastasis to ipsilateral axillary lymph node(s)
N1 = movable

N2 = fixed to one another or to the other structures

Figure 4-4: Stage III A Disease

Doctors determine how aggressively to treat and manage an individual patient based on how advanced the cancer is locally in the breast and regionally in the lymph nodes. The greater the risk of microscopic cancer cell contamination throughout the body, MICROMETASTASIS, the greater the need for treatment to destroy these undetectable cancer cells. This treatment is called ADJUVANT THERAPY because it is most often added to or administered after the surgery. Cancers proven upon initial evaluation to have spread to other organs (stage IV, METASTATIC) represent the greatest management challenge. Treatment of such cancers is referred to as METASTATIC THERAPY (see Table 4-1).

Stage 0	Ti.s.	N0	M0
Stage I	T1	N0	M0
Stage II A	T0, T1	N1	M0
	T2	N0	M0
Stage II B	T2	N1	M0
	T3	N0	M0
Stage III A	T0, T1, T2,	N2	M0
	T3	N1, N2	M0
Stage III B	Any T	N3	M0
	T4	Any N	M0
Stage IV	Any T	Any N	M1

Table 4-1: TNM Staging System

Our evolving understanding of the biology of cancer necessitates continuous revisions to the staging criteria. Subcategories have been added to provide more definition like T1a,b,c and stage IIa,b. Despite these ongoing revisions, a gap will always exist between scientific discovery and accepted policy. The clinical and pathologic findings, which fall outside of formal staging criteria but have an impact on patient outcome and the ability to predict risk of RECURRENCE, are referred to as PROGNOSTIC CRITERIA. These clinical and pathologic features are further categorized as favorable or unfavorable. Prognostic features are generally less predictive of outcome than stage and do not always stand the test of time. Some tests like FLOW CYTOMETRY FOR S-PHASE and PLOIDY (ANEOPLOID, DIPLOID-measures of DNA instability) were once commonplace but are less popular. Others like ESTROGEN RECEPTOR (ER) status and HER-2/NEU overexpression have become routine and are discussed later in this book as we turn our attention to specific breast cancer treatments. The microscopic appearance of the cancer cells has also been used as a prognostic factor. This is referred to as NUCLEAR GRADE and HISTOLOGIC GRADE. A cancer cell that retains it ductal cell features is referred to as well differentiated and grade 1. A cancer cell that retains no defining features is referred to as undifferentiated and grade 4. Grade 2 is for moderately differentiated cells, and grade 3 refers to poorly differentiated cells. Like S-phase and ploidy, nuclear grade is also falling out of favor as more specific DNA markers like Her-2/neu replace it.

I explained to Jill and Greg that her tumor was small, 1.1 cm. or T1c, but the contaminated sentinel node, N1a, resulted in her final stage of breast cancer being a stage IIa. Additionally, the cancer was estrogen sensitive or ER+, which is considered favorable. The cancer cells were also tested in the pathology laboratory to see whether they had increased amounts of the gene Her-2/neu. This was done using a screening test called the HERCEPTEST, which was intermediately positive so a confirmatory test called FLUORESCENT IN SITU HYBRIDIZATION (FISH) was performed. This test confirmed that the cancer cells had excess Her-2/neu. The amplified amounts of Her-2 were considered less favorable. In its entirety, the staging and prognostic criteria predicted that Jill had a 70% chance of being cured by her surgery or a 30% chance that she would have a relapse of this cancer during the next 10 years.

Jill and Greg were not comforted that the odds of cure were in Jill's corner. They wanted nothing less than a 100% guarantee of cure. I explained that this was not possible, but we could reduce the risk of a relapse by nearly half with adjuvant systemic therapy. We sat down for a lengthy discussion of the systemic treatment of cancer.

Systemic Therapy

The systemic theory of cancer argues that cancer is a cellular disease originating in an organ but possibly disseminated throughout the body at the time of diagnosis. If the cancer is disseminated at the time of diagnosis, then locoregional treatments would not be adequate by themselves. Systemic or total body therapies would be needed to treat the entire body in order to destroy any undetectable microscopic contaminating disease (micrometastases) or proven cancer spread (metastases).

Efforts to seek and destroy the undetectable rogue cancer cells in the circulation, or the cancer cells nesting in proven metastatic deposits, have led to the development of an arsenal of weapons—medicines that travel in the blood, poisoning cancer cells wherever they nest. Jill asked how these new medicines could cripple or destroy cancer cells. I explained how scientists examined cellular structure and function to find ways to disrupt the cancer cells' machinery.

To look at a cell in a scientific way, we would place it under a microscope. There we would see an outer cell membrane surrounding a gelatinous cytoplasm containing a nucleus at its core. Picture the Tootsie Roll Pop, as described earlier, where the wrapper is the cell membrane, the candy is the cytoplasm, and the Tootsie Roll is the nucleus. Within the nucleus is the genetic material or DNA. The DNA is a coded information system like a blueprint or an operating code (software of the cell). For a cell to live, it must continuously uncode DNA messages. Those messages are the blueprint for the production of proteins, the cells' vital machinery. Additionally, for a cell to divide and become two cells, the DNA has to be copied so that the mother cell can divide into two identical daughter cells. An effective systemic therapy would need to interfere with the DNA messages that govern cell repair, growth and division (Figure 4-5).

The very earliest forms of systemic therapy were chemicals developed to disrupt or poison DNA. The chemical agents first approved for the systemic treatment of cancer were called CHEMOTHERAPY. The logic of chemotherapy was straightforward. If cancer cells were dividing, they would have to copy their DNA to reproduce. If a treatment disrupted the DNA, the cells could not divide and could not produce daughter cells. Without daughter cells, the cancer could not grow. Furthermore, if the DNA was disrupted, the messages for the production of proteins, the cell's vital machinery that allow the cell to eat, breathe, and remove waste, could not be uncoded. If the cell could not operate its intracellular machinery, the cancer cell would die. Thus, in the-

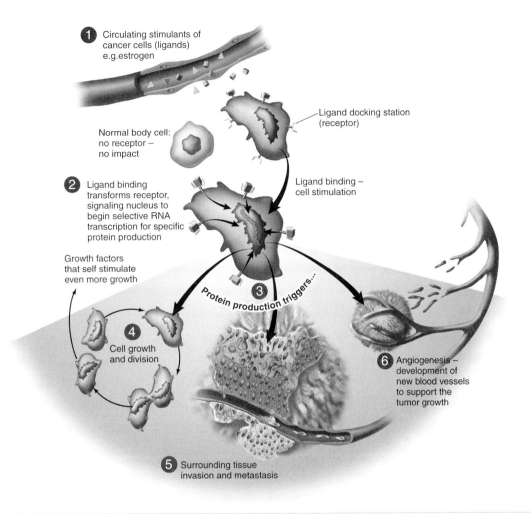

1 Circulating stimulants of cancer cells (ligands) e.g. estrogen

Ligand docking station (receptor)

Normal body cell: no receptor – no impact

Ligand binding – cell stimulation

2 Ligand binding transforms receptor, signaling nucleus to begin selective RNA transcription for specific protein production

Growth factors that self stimulate even more growth

Protein production triggers...

3

4 Cell growth and division

6 Angiogenesis – development of new blood vessels to support the tumor growth

5 Surrounding tissue invasion and metastasis

Figure 4-5: Basic Model of Systemic Therapy (An effective treatment requires interference with the processes of cancer growth and proliferation.)

ory, chemotherapy could stop the cancer growth and kill the cancer cells. Unfortunately, like cancer cells, all cells have DNA, and many cells in the body are also constantly growing and dividing: the hair cells, the blood cells, the cells that line the mouth, and the intestinal tract, etc. Therefore, these DNA-disrupting drugs (Figure 4-6) were also very toxic to normal cells.

Over the past three decades, great strides have been made to increase the effectiveness and decrease the toxicity of chemotherapy. Despite these improvements, both patients and physicians have demanded therapies that are safer, less toxic, and more cancer-cell specific. There was a call for "smart

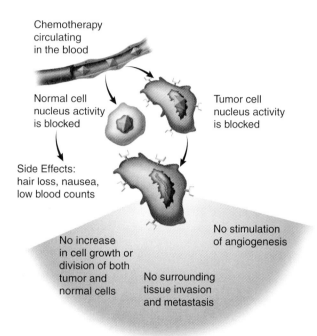

Chemotherapy
circulating
in the blood

Normal cell
nucleus activity
is blocked

Tumor cell
nucleus activity
is blocked

Side Effects:
hair loss, nausea,
low blood counts

No stimulation
of angiogenesis

No increase
in cell growth or
division of both
tumor and
normal cells

No surrounding
tissue invasion
and metastasis

Figure 4-6: How Chemotherapy Works

bombs" or "magic bullets" that could seek and destroy cancer cells without harm to the normal cell counterpart. These emerging new weapons in the arsenal against cancer have been called TARGETED THERAPY.

A cancer-specific treatment would by definition affect only cancer cells. However, these cancer cells are so genetically similar to normal cells that they escaped the recognition of the immune system. How could science accomplish what nature failed to do—target the cancer cells? The answer is in the DNA. In the past few decades, through ongoing work to translate the human genome (the basic DNA blueprint of all human cells), scientists are beginning to gain a deeper understanding of what makes a cancer cell act the way it does. With these insights, cancer management is evolving. Cancer is no longer considered an organ disease or even a cellular one. Today, cancer is considered a genetic and molecular disease. Reflecting these changes, the therapy of cancer today is not just of a cellular nature, but also one of a genetic and molecular nature.

Researchers now understand that within a given cell there are thousands of active genes (specific DNA codes) that define the cell's identity and function. These thousands of genes represent the codes for the thousands of proteins (molecules) that define the cell's structure and behavior. There may be only 1% of those genes, 1% of those important messages, that go wrong or mutate, transforming a normal cell into a cancer cell. These mutations result in the overproduction or underproduction of critical proteins that control a cell's growth and behavior and cause that cell to become malignant or cancerous. If researchers could find the 1% of those messages that are mutated, they could then target them specifically and create a magic bullet of cancer therapy. Doctors would then have a treatment that would be targeted only to the machinery gone awry in the cancer cell.

Targeted therapy may sound far fetched, but history tells us otherwise. Antibiotics were the medical magic bullets of the last century, the targeted therapy of infectious diseases. For many centuries, infection was the leading cause of death in our society. Scientists began to develop treatments for infections by first understanding the molecular differences between bacterial cells and human cells. They were then able to target specific molecules unique to the bacteria, which in turn killed the bacteria and cured the infection without harming the human host.

As it turns out, targeted therapies for cancer have been around for some time. Observations of breast cancer remission after surgical removal of the ovaries were first reported over a century ago. Although sensitivity to estrogen is not unique to mammary tissue, estrogen proved to be a powerful stimulant of some breast cancer cells. Therefore, antiestrogen therapy proved to retard the development of breast cancer while having minimal or modest effects on other normal cells of the body. This type of HORMONAL THERAPY, which has been in existence for over 40 years, really was the first targeted molecular therapy.

Today we measure the breast cancers' sensitivity to estrogen by measuring a molecule called the ESTROGEN RECEPTOR on the cancer cell surface. The receptor is metaphorically a lock that estrogen (the key or ligand) can open and in doing so stimulates the cell to grow and divide. Understanding how estrogen stimulates the cancer cell has led to a rapidly expanding arsenal of hormonal therapies. These therapies that interfere with estrogen by blocking its production or by preventing its interaction with the estrogen receptor on the cancer cell prevent estrogen's stimulatory effects; this causes sensitive cancers to go into remission. (Sensitivity to another sex hormone, PROGESTERONE, is also commonly measured; however, its predictive value is significantly less than estrogen, and therefore, it is not discussed further.)

Although this sounds so straightforward, a lot of confusion exists surrounding hormonal treatment of breast cancer, primarily because of the medical establishment's failure to speak a consistent language. Women who have been diagnosed with breast cancer are told that they cannot have or must stop hormone replacement therapy and then in the same breath are prescribed "hormonal therapy" to treat the cancer. The patient is told that she is menopausal and that she is not making estrogen, and then she is prescribed an antiestrogen therapy to block the estrogen that she was just told she is not making. Why is she given hormonal therapy when she cannot have hormones? Why is she given an antiestrogen therapy if she does not make estrogen?

Hormones are chemical messengers that are made in one part of the body and travel through the blood to other parts of the body where they have some effect. In the blood, there may be as many as a hundred distinct hormones that affect everything from menstruation, lactation, and pregnancy to metabolism and chemical balance. The hormones are categorized into groups, one of which is the sex hormones. Sex hormones are made in the ovary, testicle, and adrenal gland. Estrogen, made in the ovary, is the sex hormone that we associate with women, as its production at puberty stimulates the development of female secondary sexual characteristics; its decline in middle age signals menopause. Because the mammary tissue of the breast develops under the influence of estrogen, it is not surprising that many mammary cancers often retain estrogen sensitivity. Such an estrogen-sensitive cancer cell is stimulated to grow and divide when circulating estrogen binds to the estrogen receptors on the cell's surface (Figure 4-7).

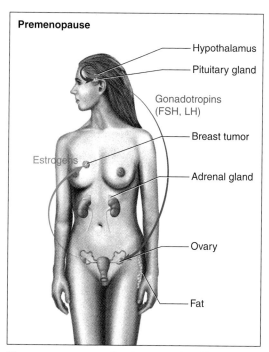

Premenopause

Hypothalamus
Pituitary gland
Gonadotropins (FSH, LH)
Breast tumor
Estrogens
Adrenal gland
Ovary
Fat

Woman: premenopausal, estrogen produced by ovary

Figure 4-7: Estrogen Receptor—Premenopausal

In a premenopausal woman, stopping that estrogen stimulation requires removing the source of estrogen, the ovary, or blocking the receptor to prevent estrogen binding. Estrogen receptors are present on many kinds of cells, not just mammary, which is why menopause has so many consequences. Scientists have tried to design drugs that will selectively block only the receptors on mammary cells. These drugs are called SELECTIVE ESTROGEN RECEPTOR MODULATORS (SERM), and two have been approved by the Food and Drug Administration: TAMOXIFEN (Nolvadex) and RALOXIFENE (Evista). Unfortunately, neither drug is perfectly selective, and thus, they still cause some unwanted SIDE EFFECTS (Figure 4-7 A, B, C, D).

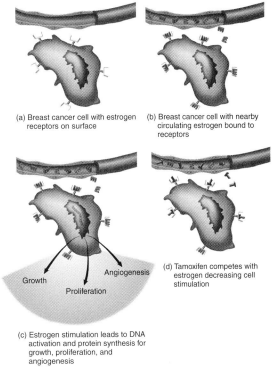

(a) Breast cancer cell with estrogen receptors on surface

(b) Breast cancer cell with nearby circulating estrogen bound to receptors

(c) Estrogen stimulation leads to DNA activation and protein synthesis for growth, proliferation, and angiogenesis

(d) Tamoxifen competes with estrogen decreasing cell stimulation

Figure 4-7 A, B, C, D: How Tamoxifen Works

As a woman approaches her fifth or sixth decade of life, the ovaries stop producing estrogen, which results in menopause and the symptoms referred to as "change of life." In truth, estrogen levels fall very low but not to zero. Although ovarian estrogen output may cease, an adrenal sex hormone is transformed into estrogen by an ENZYME found primarily in fat cells called AROMATASE. Thus, even after menopause, a woman still has some circulating estrogen. Stopping estrogen stimulation of mammary cancer cells in a postmenopausal woman thus requires either blocking the receptor with a SERM or disrupting the aromatase enzyme so that it cannot convert the adrenal hormone into estrogen. The class of drugs developed to block the aromatase reaction is called AROMATASE INHIBITORS (Figure 4-8).

Our new knowledge allows us to develop a clear and consistent language about hormones and breast cancer. The expression "estrogen replacement therapy" should replace "hormone replacement therapy." The expression "antiestrogen treatment" of breast cancer should replace "hormonal therapy" of breast cancer. Antiestrogen therapy should be further specified to identify whether that therapy is a SERM or an aromatase inhibitor.

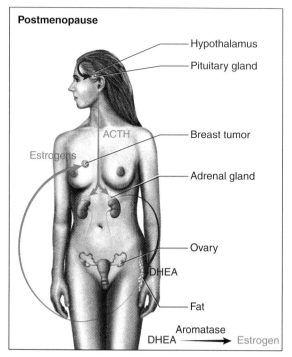

Postmenopause

Hypothalamus
Pituitary gland
ACTH
Estrogens
Breast tumor
Adrenal gland
Ovary
DHEA
Fat
Aromatase
DHEA ⟶ Estrogen

Aromatase converts androgens to estrogens in postmenopausal woman: estrogen no longer comes from ovary

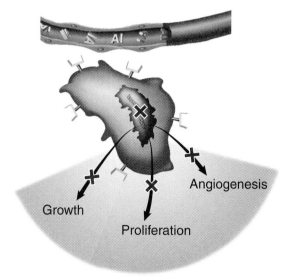

AI
Growth
Angiogenesis
Proliferation

Breast cancer cell with aromatase inhibitor in circulation preventing estrogen production–estrogen remains unbound resulting in no DNA stimulation

Figure 4-8: Estrogen Receptor–Postmenopausal   Figure 4-8 A: How Aromatase Inhibitors Work

Many breast cancer patients are advised never to take hormones because hormones could activate the cancer. In reality, they should avoid estrogen, just one of the many sex hormones in the body.

Although doctors have known about the estrogen relationship for a century and have been able to test cancer cells routinely for the estrogen receptor for over two decades, other molecular targets have been much more difficult to define. Today, over 400 molecular and genetic targets and their respective interference therapies are being investigated. The targets include receptors on the cell surface, the ligands that bind to them, the DNA which is stimulated by the transformed receptor, the RNA translation of the DNA, the proteins which the RNA define, etc. (Figure 4-9).

Thus far, one target, Her-2/neu, has resulted in a targeted therapy that has been approved for breast cancer. Scientists were interested in Her-2/neu (Her-2) because when it was activated in breast cancer cells, those cancers behaved more aggressively. A drug that has been developed to target the protein coded by the Her-2/neu gene is called HERCEPTIN. Herceptin has been proven to shrink metastases from some breast cancers that have excess or amplified amounts of the Her-2 gene. As approved by the Food and Drug Administration, Herceptin is indicated to be administered with paclitaxel chemotherapy in metastatic breast cancer patients whose tumors overexpress the Her-2 protein. Doctors now routinely study breast cancer cells to see whether they overexpress the Her-2/neu gene in order to both predict the behavior of the cancer and if the patient has metastatic breast cancer to determine whether Herceptin may be an effective therapy.

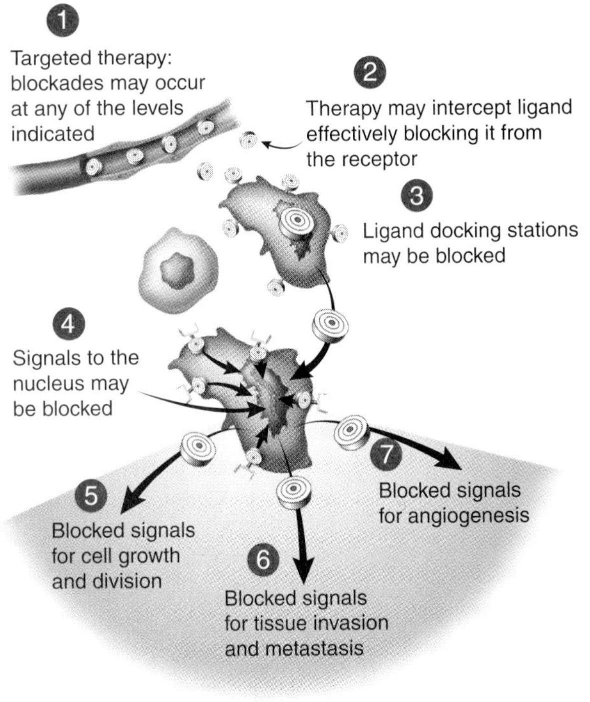

Figure 4-9: How Target Therapy Works

Today not only do doctors need to understand the tumor characteristics, the node status, and whether there is any evidence of spread to other organs of the body, but they also need to know the cancer's sensitivity to estrogen and the extent to which the cancer overproduces Her-2. All of these features have an impact on the local, regional, and systemic therapies that are recommended.

Jill and Greg were a bit overwhelmed. Her cancer was small but node positive, ER+ but Her-2 positive as well. These findings seem conflicting; small tumor and ER+ were favorable, whereas node positive and Her-2 positive were less favorable. Would Jill be required to take chemotherapy and an antiestrogen? I suggested a deep breath and counting to 10 as I took a moment to summarize what we had discussed so far. First, our understanding of cancer has evolved from the disease of an organ to a systemic cellular disease to a genetic and molecular disease. Second, there is a need for adjuvant systemic therapies in patients who are at risk for microscopic systemic contamination. Third, the staging system in conjunction with prognostic factors allows us to predict the risk of microscopic systemic contamination. Fourth, systemic therapies are of three types: chemotherapy, hormonal therapy, and the newest type of treatment, targeted therapy. Now we needed to discuss how oncologists select and integrate these treatments for each patient.

Current Treatment of Breast Cancer

Jill and Greg remained anxious as I began to explain the treatment for a stage IIa breast cancer with an involved lymph node that was both estrogen receptor positive and Her-2 amplified. When I began by explaining that there may be treatment options, they groaned. Some of the possible treatments are considered standard, whereas others would require participation in a clinical trial. Their eyes started to glaze over. I decided some background on how a standard treatment is established and what is a clinical trial might provide a better context to understand the treatment options.

For any systemic treatment to become a standard of care it must complete a long and complicated evaluation. The evaluation process incorporates three specific phases of testing: the treatment must first be proven safe (phase 1), then effective (phase 2), and then better than the current standard of care that it is replacing (phase 3). Remarkably, this process can take up to 12 years. Just as the surgical approach to the management of locoregional disease progressed over the past 30 years from the radical mastectomy to the lumpectomy with sentinel lymph node biopsy, so too has the systemic management of breast cancer evolved. This evolution occurred on two related fronts: the development of effective treatments for proven metastases and the use of those active treatments in the adjuvant setting. Effective metastatic treatments are those that reduce symptoms and prolong the life of patients with advanced cancer. Effective adjuvant treatments are those that reduce the relative risk of cancer recurrence or more simply increase the chance of cure.

The beginning of this scientific evolution can be found in the laboratory research of the late 1940s, which confirmed that certain chemicals could kill cancer cells. A decade later, the first chemotherapy drugs were administered to patients with metastatic cancer. By 1968, the chemotherapy treatment of patients with metastatic breast cancer was becoming routine. More importantly, the first reports of surgical adjuvant chemotherapy were published. Breast surgeons united to advance the science of breast cancer treatment, leading to the formation of one of the largest and most successful cooperative research organizations, the NATIONAL SURGICAL ADJUVANT BREAST AND BOWEL PROJECT (NSABP). Another decade passed before researchers could confirm that polychemotherapy (also called multidrug or combination chemotherapy) offered superior results to single-drug treatment. The first internationally recognized combination therapy was titled CMF, an acronym for the three drugs: Cytoxan, Methotrexate, and Fluorouracil.

The 1980s brought the introduction of a new class of chemotherapy drugs related to antibiotics, the ANTHRACYCLINES. The anthracycline antibiotic, ADRIAMYCIN, proved to be the most active drug to date in breast cancer therapy. Combination chemotherapy with Adriamycin (CAF/FAC) replaced CMF in metastatic disease and was increasingly used in higher risk node-positive patients. Attempts to evaluate the impact of modifications of drug doses and drug delivery schedules confirmed that 6 months of therapy were as effective as 12 months, but diluting the therapy by giving lower or less frequent doses compromised effectiveness. These studies helped to establish optimal dose and schedule, maximizing chemotherapy benefit and limiting toxicity.

The 1990s had successes and failures. A new class of chemotherapy drugs was introduced, TAXANES, with activity comparable to Adriamycin. The first targeted molecular therapy, Herceptin, was also approved. Antiestrogen therapy was advanced with the approval of aromatase inhibitors. These agents were invaluable additions to the arsenal of weapons for metastatic disease and continue to be under intense investigation in the adjuvant setting. The benefit of chemotherapy was confirmed in node-negative disease, and the additive benefit of chemotherapy plus antiestrogen therapy was proven. A new category of treatments, SUPPORT DRUGS, was introduced. These drugs have significantly improved the QUALITY OF LIFE of the cancer patient. Unfortunately, there were disappointments as well in the 1990s: highly anticipated increased cure rates with dose-intensive regimens supported by BONE MARROW stem cells, often referred to as bone marrow transplant, did not materialize.

Today, an ever-increasing volume of medical research has resulted in some very provocative phase 2 (evaluating the effectiveness of treatment) results. Unfortunately, phase 2 clinical trial results leave many unanswered questions for the patients of this new millennium: how and when to incorporate taxanes in adjuvant treatment. What is the role of the emerging arsenal of targeted therapies in the management of breast cancer and how and when should they be incorporated? Should systemic therapy be introduced after biopsy, but before definitive surgery (termed NEOADJUVANT or PRIMARY SYSTEMIC therapy)? Results from phase 2 testing, regardless of the enthusiasm with which they are reported, still require phase 3 testing for conclusive proof of superiority to warrant a change in the standard of care. Unfortunately, phase 3 testing of adjuvant treatments may take five to seven years to complete, leaving the physician and the patient to grapple with unproven options as treatment is planned.

I presented Jill and Greg with a nationally conducted, clinical study. I thought that this study represented her best option, as it not only offered her standard-of-care chemotherapy and five years of antiestrogen treatment, but also, it offered the possibility of Jill receiving an additional therapy.

Jill and Greg had to share in this important decision about participating in a clinical study. Before Jill could be enrolled, they would need to sign an informed consent document that attests to their complete understanding of all risks and benefits associated with the treatment. This was the beginning of the second most difficult job I have as a medical oncologist, explaining and comparing the risks and benefits of a clinical trial with standard treatment.

The Language of Clinical Outcomes

Understanding risks and benefits is complicated because scientists have not standardized the language of treatment-related measures and outcomes. The language of the oncologist can be very confusing. Will the doctor refer to the breast cancer as ductal, intraductal, DCIS, or noninvasive, or will he or she use all four descriptions in the same discussion? Even the word "cancer" is not uniformly used but may be substituted by malignant growth, cancerous tumor, neoplasm, etc. The outcomes of treatment are even more confusing for patients to understand as terms such as REMISSION, RESPONSE, RECURRENCE, and SURVIVAL are used to express the outcomes of therapy. Worse, for each of these outcomes like remission or response, a myriad of qualifiers will be added, including minor, partial, complete, clinical, radiographic, and pathologic. Progression and survival may be used in conjunction with or as an alternative to remission and response and then further qualified or more likely confused by qualifying descriptions such as freedom from progression, relapse-free progression, time to progression, relapse-free survival, overall survival, and disease-specific survival. If this was not confusing enough, these outcome measurements are reported as statistical probabilities, which are usually relative rather than absolute. It often sounds like double talk; how can patients and their loved ones be expected to understand? They just want to know if they will be cured.

Unbelievably, it gets worse. Many different studies are conducted on each specific treatment to prove its effectiveness and to generate outcomes, but because the study designs are not identical, the results are not either. The oncologist not only has to present this confusing data with confusing words but also he or she may have to present it for two or three studies, none of which used the same outcomes or reached the same conclusions.

After the dizzying display of data, the doctor asks the patient what he or she wants to do. The thoroughly confused patient often responds, "What would you recommend to your wife or mother?"

It does not have to be this way, and it should not. It is clear to me after nearly 20 years of caring for cancer patients that there needs to be a consensus among oncologists on how data are reported and presented to patients so that they are meaningful, the discussed risks and benefits are absolute, and the data can be compared. A researcher, Peter Ravdin, has published such an approach, and it has been made available to patients and physicians through an Internet site: *www.adjuvantonline.com*. I have begun using this simple method, which poses the question: "What would happen to 100 patients such as yourself if…." The approach is straightforward and can be quite illuminating, as my discussion with Greg and Jill illustrates. The questions Jill, Greg, and I posed were as follows: What would happen to 100 women like Jill if she did no further treatment? What would happen to 100 women like Jill if she took an antiestrogen pill only? What would happen to 100 women like Jill if she took only chemotherapy? What would happen to 100 women like Jill if she underwent chemotherapy with a sequential anthracycline plus taxane regimen and in addition underwent five years of tamoxifen treatment?

Answers to these questions are made possible by a computer analysis, which creates an age- and risk factor-adjusted assessment of cancer cure based on a huge dataset, including all relevant phase 3 clinical trials. This type of data comparison where many related but not identical clinical trials are combined is called a META-ANALYSIS and is very valuable in assessing risk for large patient populations. The dataset is further updated on a continuous basis so that the most recently completed phase 3 trials can be included in the assessment.

The analysis begins by sitting together at the computer and entering the necessary data. The online program requests information about the patient and final pathology. Jill and Greg huddled close as I typed in her age, TNM staging, and estrogen sensitivity. All that was left was to hit enter, and then the computer analysis would be under way.

The first question posed was this: Over the next 10 years, what would happen to 100 women like Jill if they chose no adjuvant systemic treatment? Studies suggest 69 women would be cured by the surgery, free of cancer. Thirty of the remaining 31 women would relapse with breast cancer metastases. One woman would die of a cause unrelated to the breast cancer. Most unfortunately, the majority of those who relapse would eventually die from the breast cancer.

The second question posed in the computer analysis was this: Over the next 10 years, what would happen to 100 women like Jill if they chose adjuvant antiestrogen therapy? Studies suggest that seven fewer women would relapse. Seventy-six women would be alive, well and free of cancer; however, 23 would have relapsed, likely to die of cancer.

The third question posed in the computer survey was this: What would happen to 100 women like Jill if adjuvant chemotherapy with a sequential anthracycline plus taxane was used? Studies suggest that the chemotherapy would save the lives of 10 women. Seventy-nine women would be alive and well, free of cancer relapse, whereas 20 women would succumb to the cancer.

The final question posed was this: Over the next 10 years, what would happen to 100 women like Jill if they chose the adjuvant chemotherapy in addition to antiestrogen therapy? The combined therapy would cure 15 more women not cured by the surgery. Eighty-four would remain alive, well and

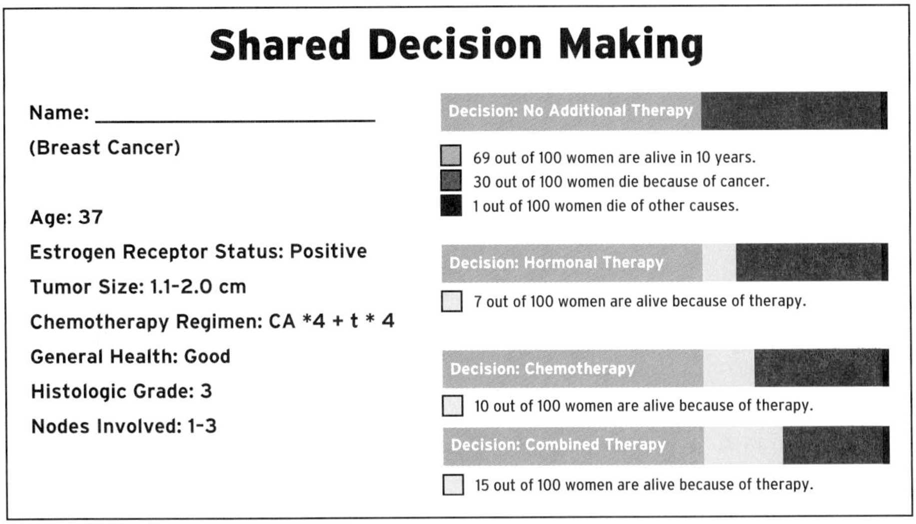

Shared Decision Making

Name: _____

(Breast Cancer)

Age: 37

Estrogen Receptor Status: Positive

Tumor Size: 1.1-2.0 cm

Chemotherapy Regimen: CA *4 + t * 4

General Health: Good

Histologic Grade: 3

Nodes Involved: 1-3

Decision: No Additional Therapy

69 out of 100 women are alive in 10 years.
30 out of 100 women die because of cancer.
1 out of 100 women die of other causes.

Decision: Hormonal Therapy

7 out of 100 women are alive because of therapy.

Decision: Chemotherapy

10 out of 100 women are alive because of therapy.

Decision: Combined Therapy

15 out of 100 women are alive because of therapy.

Figure 4-10: Adjuvantonline: Shared Decision Making

free of cancer. Only 15 women would relapse and risk cancer death. Once again one woman would die of an unrelated cause (see Figure 4-10).

An oncologist might review this information on surgery and chemotherapy and antiestrogen treatments and report that the overall cure rate is 85%, but that would not explain the specific contribution of each component of therapy (surgery, antiestrogen, chemotherapy). We might say the cure rate of adjuvant combined chemo/antiestrogen therapy is 50% because 15 of 30 women who were destined to relapse were cured. Another way this is reported is a 50% reduction in the "relative" risk of recurrence and death. It may be a more appropriate measure to say that the cure rate of chemotherapy and antiestrogen treatment is 15%, as 15 women of the 100 are cured specifically because of the combined adjuvant therapy. In other words, there is a reduction in the "absolute" risk of recurrence and death of 15%. Eight women of the 100 are cured specifically because of the contribution of chemotherapy. Is that 8% absolute improvement in cure worth the additional cost and suffering associated with the treatment? What if that benefit was only 3%? Each patient must answer that question but only with data that are clearly presented and meaningful.

When the data are presented in this way, it becomes clear that only 15 of the 100 women will truly benefit from the treatment, yet all 100 will be treated. As I explained to Jill and Greg, science has yet to develop technology that can detect micrometastases. There is no way to know who are the 69 women already cured by the surgery or who are the 15 women destined to relapse despite taking chemotherapy and antiestrogen treatment. Thus, all 100 women are treated: 69 who have no need because they are cured by surgery, 15 who have no need because it will not help, and 15 who will be truly cured by this intervention.

Jill and Greg found the discussion encouraging. Undergoing outpatient chemotherapy for four months followed by five years of tamoxifen seemed a small cost to cut in half her risk of relapse. Jill became excited when she had a sudden realization that the analysis did not include the additional therapy being studied in the clinical trial that might further increase her chance of cure. The reason that the additional therapy was not included in the analysis is that phase 3 studies evaluating its role in the adjuvant setting have not been concluded. This means that we do not currently know whether this additional therapy may benefit patients like Jill, and more importantly, we do not know what toxicities the addition may cause.

It seemed like a good time to review what we had discussed so far. The systemic therapy of cancer has evolved by demonstrating a treatment's ability to reduce the size of the cancer, prolong life, and improve care. Sequential improvements in therapy have been accomplished using a standardized three-phase approach, which confirms safety (phase 1), efficacy (phase 2), and superiority (phase 3). The process is continuous such that at any moment hundreds of research studies are ongoing in each phase. Studies not only evaluate new systemic therapies, alone and in combination, but also evaluate how to best integrate these therapies with the locoregional modalities of surgery and radiation. This dynamic and constantly improving treatment landscape may be exciting for researchers and may provide encouragement for those at risk like Jill, but it can also pose a dilemma for the patient and doctor who want to use all of the resources available to maximize the opportunity for cure and survival. Patients such as Jill and Greg, their loved ones, as well as their doctors often need some direction, some authority, to pronounce a current standard of care, define reasonable alternatives when a standard does not exist, and provide guidance for patients who wish to pursue a clinical trial option. This was my next topic of discussion with Jill and Greg.

The Standard of Care

Nationally and internationally, oncologists and cancer researchers have recognized the problems that the abundance of emerging data creates for making a treatment decision. The oncology community has responded by creating a system for peer review, discussion, and dissemination of new research. Data are released at designated meetings and in professional journals.

The oncology community has also responded by developing cooperative clinical research groups, such as the National Surgical Adjuvant Breast and Bowel Project, to provide broad patient access to new therapies in phase 2 and phase 3 testing. Consensus conferences, developed by the National Comprehensive Cancer Center Network and the National Cancer Institute, have been organized to review emerging data and to provide a consensus on patient management. The following discussions reflect those most recent consensus statements on stage-specific therapies and when and how to integrate new therapeutics into clinical practice.

DCIS

The treatment of DCIS has evolved substantially over the past decade, with the majority of women now being treated with breast-conserving surgery. The DCIS guidelines use size and extent of the lesion, grade, and margin status in identifying appropriate treatment.

Women with small (< 5 mm), low-grade, pure DCIS can be offered excision to negative margins followed by observation. This appropriate therapy is an alternative to radiation or simple mastectomy. For women with a DCIS lesion of greater than 5 mm that is not widespread, the available evidence from randomized trials demonstrates that radiation after excision to negative pathologic margins is effective. Simple mastectomy without intentional axillary lymph node removal is also considered an appropriate option. Women with widespread DCIS or with documented involvement of two or more quadrants of the breast should be treated with only simple mastectomy.

Locoregional Therapy and Stage I and Stage II Invasive Breast Cancer

Numerous trials have consistently demonstrated that modified radical mastectomy and breast conservation (complete tumor excision, axillary lymph node evaluation, and breast irradiation) are equally as effective at making patients disease free and result in equally good survival rates. A number of factors influence the choice of local therapy, including relative contraindications to breast-conserving therapy (extensive DCIS, nipple/areolar involvement, large tumor, poor cosmesis), patient preference, and available medical expertise and facilities. Other factors, such as the potential for inherited susceptibility, may also be important to discuss with patients when determining the course of therapy.

The risk of chest wall recurrence in women with primary invasive cancers greater than 5 cm or with four or more involved axillary lymph nodes is high enough that the use of postmastectomy locoregional irradiation to decrease the MORBIDITY of locoregional recurrence is recommended. Substantial controversy exists regarding the use of chest wall and regional lymph node irradiation in women postmastectomy for lesions less than 5 cm and with one to three involved axillary lymph nodes. A clinical trial in which women with one to three positive lymph nodes postmastectomy are randomized to radiation versus no radiation will hopefully resolve this issue.

Adjuvant Systemic Therapy for Stages I, II, and IIIa Invasive Breast Cancer

Estrogen and progesterone receptor content should be obtained on all primary invasive breast cancers. Patients with invasive breast cancers that are estrogen and/or progesterone receptor positive should be considered for adjuvant antiestrogen therapy. Adjuvant antiestrogen therapy is recommended in women with estrogen receptor-positive breast cancer regardless of menopausal status, age, or Her-2/neu status. Some researchers have questioned the benefit of adjuvant antiestrogen therapy in lymph node-negative cancers less than 0.5 cm or 0.6 cm or 1.0 cm and with favorable prognostic features, but the additional benefit of preventing second cancers makes the recommendation of no adjuvant antiestrogen therapy rare.

All consensus guidelines continue to recommend the use of adjuvant poly-chemotherapy (multidrugs or combination chemotherapy) in the treatment of most women with invasive breast cancer. The guidelines recommend the use of polychemotherapy in all women under 70 years of age with lymph node-positive breast cancer and with tumors greater than 1.0 cm regardless of axillary lymph node status. Guidelines recommend consideration of polychemotherapy for women with lymph node-negative breast cancer 0.6 cm to 1.0 cm in greatest di-ameter if any unfavorable features are present (unfavorable features include an-giolymphatic invasion, high S-phase, high nuclear grade, high histologic grade, Her-2 over expression, and estrogen receptor negative).

Selection of Optimal Adjuvant Systemic Therapy

All patients with estrogen receptor-positive tumors should receive antiestro-gen treatment for five years. Premenopausal patients should be offered oophorectomy or tamoxifen. Postmenopausal patients should receive treat-ment with an aromatase inhibitor. Patients with estrogen receptor-negative tumors should not be offered adjuvant therapy with an antiestrogen.

The treatment of choice for patients with estrogen receptor-negative tumors is combination chemotherapy, preferably with an anthracycline-containing regimen. Low-risk patients, those with small tumors (T1), no lymph node involvement (N0), and favorable prognostic factors (ER+, Her-2-negative), may receive equal benefit from either an abbreviated four-cycle course of the anthracycline regimen AC and the older, less toxic regimen CMF. The multidrug regimens (FAC, CAF, FEC, or CEF) are pre-ferred for higher risk patients who have tumors greater than 2 cm or who are node positive or who have unfavorable prognostic features. Six cycles of ther-apy with a single regimen are probably optimal. The addition of taxanes should be considered for all high-risk patients with lymph node-positive breast cancer, especially if the cancer is estrogen receptor negative. Prelimi-nary response and survival data suggest that anthracycline plus taxane either concurrently or in sequence may represent the optimal therapy in appropri-ately selected high-risk patients. For most patients at intermediate or high risk of recurrence and with estrogen receptor-positive tumors, the sequential administration of combination chemotherapy followed by antiestrogen ther-apy for five years is the treatment of choice. The improved outcomes achieved with aromatase inhibitors over tamoxifen in postmenopausal women suggest that those women already receiving tamoxifen in the adjuvant setting should consider changing to an aromatase inhibitor or sequentially taking an aromatase inhibitor for at least two years after completion of their five-year tamoxifen therapy.

Optimally performed interventions provide maximal benefits. Chemotherapy is no substitute for good surgery or vice versa. The combined use of optimal surgery, chemotherapy, antiestrogen therapy, and radiotherapy has a major impact on the risk of recurrence.

Jill and Greg found the discussion and informed consent a bit overwhelming. They decided that their best treatment option was a combination chemotherapy program in which a four-cycle course of Adriamycin and Cytoxan would be followed in sequence by a four-cycle course of a taxane. Based on our discussions and their own research, this combination offered the best reduction in recurrence risk that could be achieved with chemotherapy. After chemotherapy, antiestrogen therapy consisting of a five-year course of a daily antiestrogen pill (tamoxifen, because Jill is premenopausal) would further reduce the risk of a relapse. Jill and Greg were puzzled that this plan did not include Herceptin, even though her cancer was likely sensitive, as it overexpressed the Her-2 protein. I explained that Herceptin, like the other emerging targeted therapies, is a relatively new anticancer therapy. Phase 3 testing of new therapeutics is first performed in patients with more advanced disease than Jill's. Although Herceptin proved effective in phase 3 testing in metastatic patients, leading to its approval by the Food and Drug Administration and its place in the arsenal of systemic therapies used in the care of patients with metastatic disease, phase 3 testing in the adjuvant setting would need to be successfully completed before it could be used for patients with more limited cancer like Jill. The clinical trial that Jill and Greg had reviewed was addressing the very question of whether adding an additional therapy to a standard chemotherapy and antiestrogen therapy in women with node-positive breast cancer might further reduce the risk of recurrence without unacceptable toxicity.

After a bit more deliberation, participating in the clinical trial seemed like a reasonable solution to all of Jill's concerns, but Greg seemed hesitant. He was concerned that she might enroll in the trial but not receive the additional therapy. Greg was correct. In order to prove that a therapeutic drug adds benefit, clinical trials are structured so that some of the patients receive the current standard of care, whereas others receive the standard treatment plus the therapeutic drug under investigation. This kind of trial design is the most common and is referred to as RANDOMIZED, where patients are randomly assigned to receive either the standard treatment arm or the arm evaluating the risk/benefit of the additional therapy. Jill did not understand why I just could not give her the standard treatment plus the additional therapy because she knew another patient in my office was getting it and was not on a clinical trial. Giving therapies to patients before they are approved is risky, as clinical trials not only evaluate the reduction in risk of recurrence but also the negative aspects of new therapies, such as side effects and complications. The only way Jill could receive an investigational therapy was by participation in a clinical trial and only then if randomized to the investigational arm.

After one more night to sleep on their decision, Jill and Greg signed the informed consent. The following Monday, after all necessary tests were completed per the clinical trial requirements, treatment was begun. Blood tests, additional x-rays, and a test to measure her heart function had been performed, and fortunately, no abnormalities were detected. Jill was randomized to receive the investigational-additional therapy as well as the chemotherapy and Tamoxifen.

Over the subsequent weeks more questions arose. Jill's mother accompanied Jill to the clinic one day to discuss breast cancer prevention. On another occasion, Jill and Greg wanted to know how I would know Jill was in remission or relapse. There were also questions about monitoring Jill after she finished her treatments (these questions are addressed in Chapter 5). The most difficult question arose after Jill and Greg read an article about a new treatment for breast cancer that appeared superior to what she was receiving. The treatment was called "Dose Dense," and it differed from prior treatment strategies by delivering the chemotherapy at closer intervals. Rather than the chemotherapy drugs being administered every three weeks, as Jill was receiving them, they were given every two weeks. Support medicines were needed to permit such rapid chemotherapy scheduling, making the treatment very expensive but no more toxic.

I explained that the "Dose Dense" concept and the results of the clinical trial testing the concept were both very exciting, but they also may be considered preliminary. The average patient enrolled in the trial had only been under surveillance for three years, and some of the outcomes were controversial, such as the absence of some commonly seen complications. The real proof of principle with such concepts happens when the trial is repeated and the results are confirmed and when patient outcomes are measured at 5 and 10 years. They were much more comforted when I explained that women who enrolled in this trial were not offered the additional therapy.

The "Dose Dense" discussion raised the broader question of how a patient and her supportive family members remain sane amidst the endless reports of breakthroughs, miracles, and cures. There is no easy answer. In my observation, the key to sanity can be found in a patient's trust in the integrity of her caregiver and faith in her own judgment. All patients will reach a line in the sand when they have to decide on treatment. Only by believing that they have performed adequate due diligence and by trusting their caregiver's recommendations can that decision be made without regret. Jill and Greg went through such a process. I believe they had a foundation of faith and trust that would keep them sane in the coming months and years.

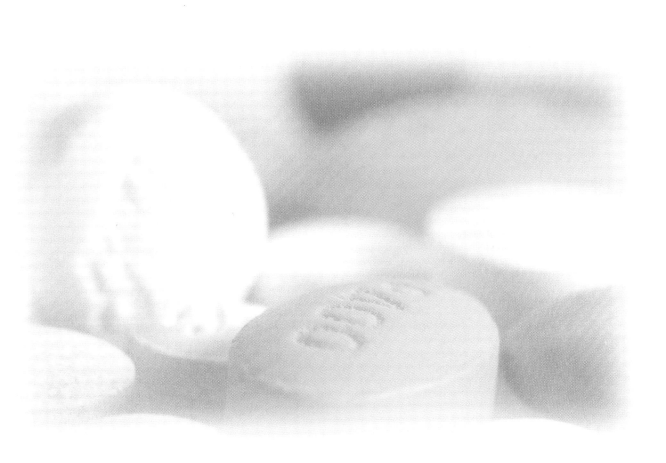

SECTION 3

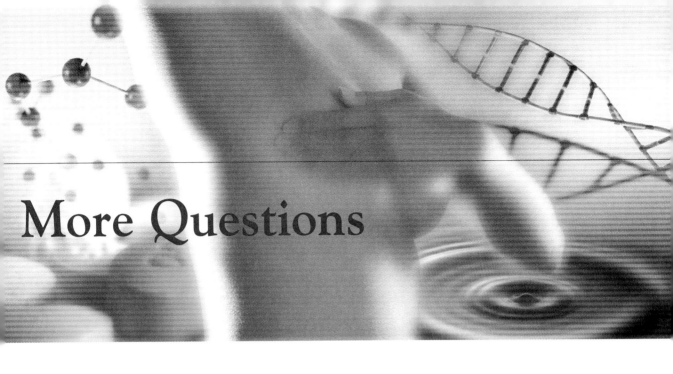

More Questions

Chapter Five

Alternative Therapies

Jill and Greg raised the possibility of pursuing alternative therapy. Thankfully, before embarking on such an initiative, they consulted with me. I thought some definitions were needed to help us structure the discussion. Unconventional, alternative, or complementary therapies encompass a broad spectrum of practices and beliefs and are, therefore, very difficult to define. What is common to these therapies is that they are not in conformity with the beliefs or standards of the conventional mainstream medical establishment or accepted standard of care. These standards can also be culturally dependent, which may create further confusion. Traditional Chinese medicine is considered unconventional in the United States, whereas it is a standard practice in China. Also, with unconventional therapies, their proof of effectiveness is most often conveyed through personal anecdote rather than stringent evidence-based criteria reached through multiphase clinical research.

Unconventional therapies may be subdivided into COMPLEMENTARY THERAPIES and ALTERNATIVE THERAPIES. Complementary therapies can be further categorized as spiritual, psychological, nutritional, and physical. Meditation, relaxation, imaging, prayer, massage, and dietary supplements would be just a few of the interventions included in this vital quartet of complementary therapies. These approaches to healing are not in conflict with conventional Western medicine; rather, in most cases, they can be effectively integrated into standard medical practice. Alternative therapies, as the name implies, are not intended to be integrated into conventional therapy; rather, they are offered as a complete therapy. Unproven by evidence-based criteria, pharmacologic treatments comprise the bulk of alternative therapies. These therapies are particularly susceptible to quackery, and false and excessive claims and high-profit motives are common.

The increased interest in and attractiveness of unconventional therapies are understandable. The technologic and frequently impersonal nature of modern medicine leaves patients feeling lost and empty. Insensitive, hurried interactions with physicians often result in patients feeling helpless, out of control, and ignored. The confusing jargon and statistics further alienate the patient and family. Finally, the cold, hard truth of some cancer diagnoses and the limited effectiveness of some conventional standard therapies may foster hopelessness. Unconventional medicine, on the other hand, is perceived as natural, simpler, nontoxic, and more understandable. Its practitioners are viewed as more caring and their approach more holistic. The absence of data eliminates the difficult discussions of toxicity, response, and survival probability.

Greg asked, "How does one evaluate and choose an unconventional approach to healing?"

There are a few guidelines that I suggest my patients follow. First, avoid any practitioner of any unconventional (or for that matter mainstream) method who is evasive. People who are practicing healing techniques that they believe in will want to share them with your other doctors, not hide them. Second, avoid treatments that are touted to work only if you stop your traditional treatments. Especially with cancer treatment, we need to take advantage of *all* treatments that may help. Third, avoid practitioners who have exclusive access to the cure but will not tell anyone what it is. Practitioners who truly believe in what they are doing want to share their successes. Fourth, beware of the motivations of the people making recommendations. It is unusual for natural healing techniques to be very expensive. If an exclusive treatment is being suggested and is very expensive, examine the motivations of the prescriber. Be aware that most unconventional therapies are not covered by insurance, given the absence of supporting data from well-designed clinical trials. Finally, pick an unconventional therapy that you feel good enough about to discuss with your physician. Your participation in restoring or maintaining your health is absolutely essential. The success of many alternative treatments depends in great part on your belief in the potential of the therapy to improve your health. If you truly believe in the therapy, be willing to discuss it not only with your family and friends, but also with your physician.

Jill and Greg seemed comfortable with my response. I told them that if they came across a particularly appealing complementary treatment to bring it to my attention for discussion. As I was about to leave the room, I noticed Jill appeared uneasy. I asked again if she was comfortable with her decision. She said that this was not what was troubling her. She said she worried about her mom's risk of breast cancer even though she tested negative for the BRCA gene. I told her that there were steps her mom could take right now to reduce her risk of getting breast cancer.

Prevention

Strategies have recently been designed that may help to prevent first and subsequent breast cancers. These strategies include lifestyle modifications, genetic testing, surgery, and medicine. Diet and exercise may play an important role in prevention. Dietary fats, alcohol, sedentary behavior, and obesity are all being investigated as possible factors that increase risk of cancer. Studies of both men and women have suggested that three or more hours of vigorous exercise a week may significantly reduce the risk of developing cancer. Dietary fats have been thought to be related to breast cancer because countries with very low breast cancer incidence, for example Japan, also have very low-fat diets. Unfortunately, this remains unproven, as research has failed to test diets as low in fats (15%) as those followed in Asia and Africa. Alcohol's effect on the liver may increase circulating estrogen levels, which is why its relationship to breast cancer incidence is under investigation.

A great deal of research has also been focused on developing drugs that can prevent cancer. The preventative treatment of cancer with a drug is called CHEMOPREVENTION. One drug, called tamoxifen (Nolvadex), has now been approved for the chemoprevention of breast cancer. Tamoxifen is now being tested against a second drug called raloxifene (Evista) to see whether raloxifene may be equally effective in prevention or possibly even superior or with fewer side effects. Early research suggests that breast cancers may be reduced by as much as 50% with medications that interfere with estrogen. Who should receive chemoprevention, with what drug, and for how long remains to be established, but multidisciplinary consensus conferences using evidence-based clinical research are beginning to shed light on this area.

A community survey found that 23% of women expressed interest in breast cancer chemoprevention. Worry about breast cancer was the strongest predictor of interest, but there was no association between interest and objec-

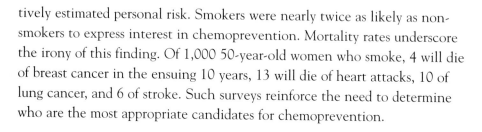

tively estimated personal risk. Smokers were nearly twice as likely as non-smokers to express interest in chemoprevention. Mortality rates underscore the irony of this finding. Of 1,000 50-year-old women who smoke, 4 will die of breast cancer in the ensuing 10 years, 13 will die of heart attacks, 10 of lung cancer, and 6 of stroke. Such surveys reinforce the need to determine who are the most appropriate candidates for chemoprevention.

Doctors welcome the latest recommendations for chemoprevention of breast cancer from the U.S. Preventive Services Task Force (USPSTF). The recommendations are based on the four clinical trials that have addressed the use of selective estrogen receptor modulators, specifically tamoxifen and raloxifene, for primary prevention of breast cancer.

The largest trial, conducted with high-risk women, was the National Surgical Adjuvant Breast and Bowel Project P-1 Study, known as the Breast Cancer Prevention Trial (BCPT). The BCPT was terminated early after finding a relative reduction in breast cancer incidence of 49% and an absolute risk reduction of just over 20 cases per 1,000 women taking tamoxifen over five years. The effect was limited to estrogen receptor-positive tumors.

The Multiple Outcomes of Raloxifene Evaluation trial, which was not limited to high-risk women, found breast cancer incidence to be 76% lower with raloxifene than with PLACEBO, with an absolute risk reduction of 8 cases per 1,000 women over 40 months. Again, the effect was limited to estrogen receptor-positive tumors.

The Royal Marsden Hospital Chemoprevention Trial and the Italian Tamoxifen Prevention Study compared tamoxifen with placebo but failed to find a reduction in breast cancer incidence. However, the use of exogenous estrogen (estrogen replacement therapy) was allowed in the European trials but not in the BCPT, and the duration of tamoxifen therapy was longer in the BCPT, raising doubts about the conclusions in these European studies.

On the basis of this review of the evidence, the USPSTF recommends against widespread use of chemoprevention for patients with a low or average risk for breast cancer. The USPSTF recommends discussing chemoprevention with selected patients at high risk for breast cancer and at low risk for the most serious adverse events (endometrial cancer, pulmonary embolus, and stroke induced by tamoxifen), (see Table 2-1, page 27).

The current evidence leaves many questions unanswered. Do chemoprevention agents prevent cancer or treat very early cases? How long does the effect of lowered incidence of breast cancer persist after taking a chemopreventive drug for five years? Will breast cancer cells develop resistance to tamoxifen? Together, these issues beg the big question: does chemoprevention reduce breast cancer and all-cause mortality and, if so, by how much?

The USPSTF recommendations present two serious challenges for clinicians. First, clinicians must respond to the misinformed and mitigate the worry that may cloud perspective and create demand for chemoprevention when the potential harms far exceed the benefits. Second, clinicians must identify and engage the uninformed for whom, because of their risk profile and personal preference, chemoprevention holds potential promise.

Risk estimation and communication are at the center of both challenges. The most frequently used risk assessment tool, the Gail Model, estimates the five-year incidence of breast cancer for a patient on the basis of the woman's age, number of first-degree relatives with breast cancer, no pregnancies, or age at birth of first child, number of breast biopsies, pathologic diagnosis of atypical hyperplasia, and age at menarche. For women whose worry results from an exaggerated perception of risks, such estimates may provide reassurance.

Making fateful decisions that depend on medical science as well as highly personal judgments about how future illness will affect quality of life is difficult at best. Neither doctor nor patient can do it alone. With breast cancer chemoprevention, clinicians and patients need to understand the limits of what we know and what we can control about the future. Women and doctors who work at making good decisions together will be far more likely to make the best use of what current medical science has to offer. After much thought, Jill and her mom decided that five years of tamoxifen might not be the best choice for her mom. We all agreed that it was appropriate to continue annual mammography and her daily two-mile walk. Jill's mom also agreed to limit her wine consumption to the weekends and increase the amount of fruits and vegetables in her diet.

Chapter Seven

Advanced Cancer

Jill and Greg had raised the "what if" question about relapse. I had hoped to avoid this discussion as it can be unpleasant to talk about treatment failure which was unlikely given Jill's probability of cure. Occasionally, cancer will recur only in the preserved breast, axilla, or chest wall. In these cases, it is referred to as a LOCAL RECURRENCE and is likely curable. However, most relapses are systemic, which means they are metastases. Metastases are rarely cured. I could not think of a gentle way to approach metastatic cancer and thus I decided to detour for a bit, beginning the discussion with locally advanced cancer, a subject that I neglected in our earlier discussion.

Locally Advanced High-Risk Breast Cancer

I have previously focused on women who undergo surgical removal of the breast tumor and subsequent adjuvant therapy to destroy micrometastasis and reduce the risk of relapse. These women are said to have LOCALIZED breast cancer, and consensus guidelines offer reasonable clarity in the approach to management. I now discuss the woman with locally advanced breast cancer: either a large breast mass (greater than 5 cm) or palpable auxiliary lymph nodes at presentation or a breast mass that involves the overlying skin or is fixed to the underlying chest wall. Guidelines to direct management of these patients is less clear, and thus, I will share where current research is leading us.

A woman who presents with locally advanced breast cancer may benefit from a new treatment approach—chemotherapy before surgery. This approach, called neoadjuvant chemotherapy (or primary systemic therapy), attempts to make the cancer more accessible to breast conservation surgery.

Unlike with chemotherapy in the adjuvant setting—which treats possible micrometastases—the effect of neoadjuvant chemotherapy can be directly observed as either the tumor shrinks, remains stable, or grows. Recent studies demonstrate growth of tumor during treatment in less than 10% of neoadjuvantly treated patients. Neoadjuvant chemotherapy demonstrates the effectiveness of chemotherapy (chemo sensitivity) and shrinks tumors, permitting breast conservation. These benefits as well as the hope that such an approach may increase the cure rate in this high-risk population are making the neoadjuvant approach increasingly popular among physicians and patients. Regardless of the approach, the successful treatment of women with locally advanced breast cancer requires the coordinated efforts of a surgical, radiation, and medical oncologist. All three treatment modalities are needed to optimize the cure rate.

Metastatic Breast Cancer

The evaluation of patients with metastatic disease either at initial presentation or after relapse can be performed in a similar way. Unfortunately, cure is rare in metastatic disease, and thus, the important measure is survival time. I recommend using the percentage of women alive at 1, 2, 3, or 5 years after treatment as a meaningful measure of treatment effectiveness. Survival may be the ultimate goal of treatment, but the care of the patient with metastatic disease is complicated by the need to manage disease-related symptoms. Before survival can be considered, suffering must be palliated. The ability of a treatment to palliate symptoms is measured as its response rate. Response may be more important than survival in a suffering patient. Outcomes, such as one-year survival and clinical response, are most commonly presented in relative terms but can also be presented as absolute impact in the 100-patient method.

Despite all of the described methods to screen, diagnose, and adjuvantly treat breast cancer when it is localized, 25% of all breast cancer patients still die from their disease because the cancer metastasizes to the vital organs: lung, liver, and brain. They also may suffer from cancer involvement of bone, lymph nodes, and skin, and recurrences take place in the chest wall of the originally involved breast. Breast cancer in this setting is rarely curable, but a great deal can be done to diminish symptoms, improve quality of life, and prolong life. Therapy intended not to cure but to improve the quality of life is called PALLIATIVE.

Because all treatments have side effects, palliative therapy demands a uniquely candid discussion of goals and objectives between the oncologist and patient. Expressions such as "watch and wait," "the cure may be worse than the disease," and "win the battle but lose the war" are attempts by oncologists to explain to the patient that when it comes to palliative therapy, more is not always better. The main objective in palliative therapy is maximal preservation of quality of life, not maximal tumor shrinkage, unless shrinkage (response) has been proven to impact directly the quality of life or survival.

Chapter Eight

Posttreatment Surveillance

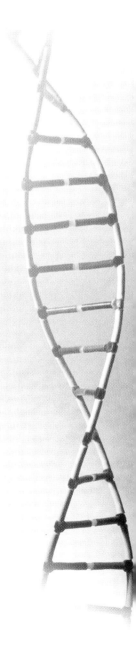

onsensus panels continue to recommend posttreatment follow-up for women with Stages I, II, and III breast cancer. Follow-up should include performance of routine history and physical examinations, mammography, and, if treated with tamoxifen, pelvic examination if the uterus is present. Surveillance may be as frequent as every three months in the first few years after diagnosis or as infrequent as annually beyond five years from diagnosis. However, surveillance is recommended for the life of the patient as both late relapse of breast cancer and late adverse effects of treatments have been reported as many as 30 years after diagnosis. Routine surveillance by BONE SCAN and CT SCAN are not recommended to the dismay of most patients. Unfortunately, neither of these approaches has been proven effective. Similar to the screening tests that were discussed earlier, for a surveillance method to be effective, it must be proven to be both sensitive and specific. Insensitive tests will miss abnormalities. Sensitive tests that are not specific will reveal abnormalities that are not related to the cancer, often leading to more tests, procedures, and anxiety that may not only be not helpful but seriously harmful. Researchers continue to evaluate new technologies that might enhance the ability to both diagnose and predict relapse. PET scanning and other imaging and genetic and routine blood chemistry testing such as the CA 27-29 and CA 15-3 are still considered investigational. Genomics and proteinomics as well as microarray testing hold the greatest promise but may not be commercially available until the close of the decade.

Epilogue

During the next few months, Jill and Greg slowly settled into the reality of her therapy. The first six weeks were the toughest, as she experienced reconstruction-related pain, suffered the indignity of hair loss, and dealt with the side effects of chemotherapy. The emotional impact of her treatment overwhelmed her more than the physical effects. It's not easy to confront mortality at any age, certainly not at thirty-seven. Greg and the kids' doting and well-intentioned support only worsened her sense of vulnerability. She became clinically depressed. I recommended counseling and an antidepressant. She agreed.

Three months into systemic therapy, Jill seemed to turn a corner. Counseling and antidepressant therapy were helping. Her treatment tolerance improved and the reconstruction-related pain resolved. She was mostly bothered by a sense of fatigue that she likened to that experienced during her pregnancies. Now, Jill was finally able to look at herself in the mirror without becoming ill and crying. She was beginning to feel that the worst was behind her and that life might return to normal.

Near the conclusion of chemotherapy, she experienced an emotional setback. I thought she would approach the day of her last treatment with elation, but surprisingly, she seemed depressed. Our conversation uncovered a growing emotional dependency on her active treatment as her protection against a cancer relapse. I explained that her chemotherapy had accomplished what was intended and that it was time to advance her treatment to antiestrogen therapy. The five years of oral tamoxifen, which she was about to initiate, was as important to her cure as was the chemotherapy. She started taking tamoxifen, remaining upbeat and resilient despite the severe hot flashes that would continue for three months.

Two years from that fateful day when the words "you have cancer" forever changed their lives, Jill, Greg, Amy, and Josh were a happy and healthy suburban family once again. Selective memory and the healing effects of time proved to be an effective salve to the physical and emotional wounds inflicted by her cancer diagnosis. Like millions of Americans, Jill and Greg found that they had what it takes to be survivors.

My only remaining question as I close this discussion of breast cancer answers is on the lighter side: did I have what it takes to survive a classroom of fifteen second-graders? As you recall, I left Daniel's room contemplating what kind of cancer machine to demonstrate and what memento I could leave for the class. I decided Legos were a more than adequate prop for my presentation. After all, a two-ton linear accelerator would not fit through the classroom door.

What to give second-graders was a bigger challenge. I contacted Ken, a pharmaceutical representative, who said he could donate some promotional fanny-packs. His company's marketing department developed the fanny-pack filled with exercise-related items including a water bottle, towel, and stopwatch to create the notion that the fatigue-busting drug for cancer patients could get them back into exercising. I was elated as I realized that a fanny-pack bulging with all this junk would be the best give-away that any parent could have.

The day arrived, and before curious eyes, Daniel and I entered the classroom with Legos and fanny-packs. Daniel's teacher brought the class to order, then asked Daniel to introduce me.

Daniel's introduction was the essence of brevity. "This is my dad."

The kids were great. They were attentive, well behaved and—believe it or not—interested. Upon the conclusion of my demonstration, the teacher asked the students if they had any questions. The hands shot up. I was overwhelmed at the response and pointed to a boy in the back row. He asked, "What's the best thing about your job?" I said, "It's nice to be able to help people." More hands soared. "What's the worst part of your job?" I explained that I'm not able to make all the sick people who see me feel better. More hands went up, and my head was swelling to the size of a watermelon. "What's the best part of your job?" I said, "In addition to helping people I get to come home at night and play with Daniel." I looked at Daniel; he was beaming. More hands. "What's the worst part of your job?" I may be gullible, but I'm not stupid. "Is there anyone with a question other than what is the best or worst part of my job?" I was praying that just one hand would still be up, but none were. They were all shills asking the questions planted by their teacher.

Once again, I was humbled by children. I thanked the teacher and said good-bye to the class. As I left, I looked over my shoulder to see Daniel grinning ear to ear.

Glossary

Acquired mutations: genetic alterations resulting from chronic physical, chemical, radiation, and natural injury to DNA; responsible for 90% of adult malignancy.

Adenocarcinoma: a form of cancer that develops from a malignant transformation of the cells lining a glandular organ such as the breast; almost all breast cancers are adenocarcinomas.

Adjuvant therapy: an additional treatment used to increase the effectiveness of the primary therapy; chemotherapy is often used as an adjuvant treatment after a mastectomy.

Adriamycin: the most commonly used anthracycline antibiotic-type chemotherapy.

Alternative therapies: unconventional cancer therapies offered as replacement to standard modalities of chemotherapy and radiation; not recognized by medical establishment or insurers, often untested but supported by personal anecdote.

Amino acids: specific types of chemical compounds that are the building blocks of proteins.

Aneuploid: having an abnormal number of sets of chromosomes; for example, tetraploid means having two paired sets of chromosomes, which is twice as many as normal; aneuploid cancer cells tend not to respond as well to therapy; aneuploidy refers to the state of being aneuploid; see also diploid and ploidy.

Angiogenesis: the growth of new blood vessels, a characteristic of tumors; angiogenesis is a normal biologic process that occurs in both healthy and diseased states; "angiogenesis factor" or "tumor angiogenesis factor" refers to a substance that tumors produce in order to grow new blood vessels.

Anthracycline antibiotic: a class of chemotherapy drugs; the most common brand names include Adriamycin, Epirubicin, and Doxil.

Aromatase: an enzyme that converts an adrenal chemical to estrogen (estradiol or estrone), primarily found in fat cells but also found in muscle and liver cells.

Aromatase inhibitor: a drug that blocks an enzyme that converts an adrenal chemical to estrogen (estradiol or estrone).

Aspiration: the use of suction to remove fluid or tissue, usually through a fine needle (e.g., aspiration biopsy).

Atypical ductal hyperplasia: a precancerous overgrowth of duct cells.

Axilla: the anatomic name for the armpit.

Axillary dissection: the surgical evaluation of the axillary (armpit) by opening the axillary fascia and removing lymph nodes along the axillary vein.

Axillary sampling: removal of some axillary nodes without a required or formal entry of axillary fascia and dissection along the axillary vein.

Benign: relatively harmless; not cancerous; not malignant.

Bilateral: both sides; for example, a bilateral mastectomy is a mastectomy in which both breasts are removed.

Biopsy: sampling of tissue from a particular part of the body (e.g., the breast) in order to check for abnormalities such as cancer; removed tissue is typically examined microscopically by a pathologist in order to make a precise diagnosis of the patient's condition.

Bone marrow: soft tissue in bone cavities that produces blood cells.

Bone scan: a technique that is more sensitive than conventional x-rays, it uses a radio labeled agent to identify abnormal or cancerous growths within or attached to bone; in the case of breast cancer, a bone scan is used to identify bone metastases; metastases appear as "hot spots" on the film; however, the absence of hot spots does not prove the absence of tiny metastases.

BRCA: a mutated gene associated with breast cancer. Types 1 and 2 can be routinely tested in high-risk women.

Breast-conservation surgery: a surgical procedure in which the cancer is removed, but the breast is spared; also called segmental mastectomy, quadrantectomy, and lumpectomy.

Breast ultrasound: a sound or sonar evaluation of the breasts useful when mammogram is not equivocal, especially in young women.

Cancer: the growth of abnormal cells in the body in an uncontrolled manner; unlike benign tumors, cancerous tumors tend to invade surrounding tissues and spread to distant sites of the body via the bloodstream and lymphatic system.

Carcinogenesis: the sequential genetic and molecular changes that are responsible for cellular transformations into cancer.

Carcinoma: a form of cancer that originates in organ tissues as a result of transformation of the epithelial cells.

Chemoprevention: the use of a pharmaceutical or other substance to prevent the development of cancer.

Chemotherapy: the use of pharmaceuticals or other chemicals to kill cancer cells; in many cases, chemotherapeutic agents kill not only cancer cells but also other cells in the body, making such agents potentially very dangerous.

Chromosome: a thread-like linear strand of DNA and associated proteins in the nucleus of cells that carries the genes and functions in the transmission of hereditary information.

Clinical trial: a carefully planned experiment to evaluate a treatment or a medication (often a new pharmaceutical) for an unproven use; phase 1 trials are very preliminary short-term trials involving a few patients designed to evaluate safety; phase 2 trials may involve 20 to 50 patients and are designed to estimate the most active dose of a new drug and evaluate efficiency; phase 3 trials involve many patients and compare a new therapy against the current standard or best available therapy to evaluate superiority.

Complementary therapies: unconventional therapies that can be effectively integrated into standard medical care but not necessarily endorsed by the medical establishment or proven to improve outcomes by evidence-based criteria.

Complete axillary node dissection: the removal of all (approximately 40) axillary lymph nodes by dissecting along the axillary vein below (level 1), under (level 2), and above (level 3) the pectoralis muscle (also see axillary dissection).

Complete response: total disappearance of all evidence of disease; when disease is no longer detected using physical examination, laboratory studies, and radiologic imaging; a criterion for evaluating the efficacy of a particular anticancer therapy (see partial response).

Complication: an unexpected or unwanted effect of a treatment, pharmaceutical, or other procedure.

Computerized axial tomography (CAT or CT scan): a method of combining images from multiple x-rays under the control of a computer to produce cross-sectional or three-dimensional pictures of the internal organs that can be used to identify abnormalities; used for evaluating metastases of the lymph nodes or more distant soft tissue sites.

Congenital mutations: gene alterations that develop in utero.

Core biopsy: the removal of a core of tissue from a tumor for the purpose of pathologic examination.

CT scan: computerized or computed tomography (CAT scan).

Diagnosis: the evaluation of signs, symptoms, and selected test results by a physician to determine the physical and biological causes of the signs and symptoms and whether a specific disease or disorder is involved.

Differentiation: (1) the process by which the homogenous cells of the developing embryo change into the 200+ cell types of the human being and the process showing how mature (developed) the cancer cells are in a tumor; (2) differentiated tumor cells resemble normal cells and grow at a slower rate than undifferentiated tumor cells, which lack the structure and function of normal cells and grow more aggressively.

Diploid: having one complete set of normally paired chromosomes, that is, a normal amount of DNA; a diploid number of chromosomes would equal 46, and a haploid set would equal 23 (also see ploidy).

DNA: the basic biologically active chemical that defines the physical development and growth of nearly all living organisms; a complex protein that is the carrier of genetic information.

Duct: the tube-like structure of mammary tissue that transfers mothers' milk from the lobule cells to the nipple.

Ductal carcinoma: a nonspecific term used to describe cancer of mammary tissue.

Ductal carcinoma in situ: the earliest form of breast cancer before it invades through the duct wall.

Ductal hyperplasia: the earliest change of duct cell growth, characterized by orderly overgrowth.

Ectoderm: the layer of pre-embryologic cells that gives rise to skin and nerves.

Electromagnetic spectrum: the range of radiant energy that is distinguished by wavelength and includes therapeutic radiation, visible light, radiowaves, etc.

Embryo: the human in its earliest stage of intrauterine development.

Endoderm: the layer of cells in the developing embryo that gives rise to the body's organs.

Enzyme: any of a group of chemical substances that are produced by living cells and that cause particular chemical reactions to happen while not being changed themselves.

Epithelial cell: those cells derived from the endoderm and that comprise the organs.

Estrogen: a sex hormone associated with female secondary sex characteristics.

Estrogen receptor: the docking site on the cell for estrogen. It is a protein that can be measured and quantified.

Excisional biopsy: the removal of an area of diseased tissue in its entirety for submission for pathologic review.

External beam radiation therapy: a form of radiation therapy in which the radiation is delivered by a machine directed at the area to be radiated as opposed to radiation given within the target tissue such as brachytherapy.

Fine-needle aspiration: removal of cellular material from diseased tissue via a needle for submission for pathologic review.

Flow cytometry: a measurement method that determines the fraction of cells that are diploid, tetraploid, aneuploid, etc. (ploidy status), as well as the percent of DNA undergoing synthesis (S-phase).

Fluorescent in situ hybridization: a laboratory technique that can identify specific DNA sequences.

Fraction: the portion of a fractionated radiation treatment that is delivered in a single session.

Gamma radiation: very short wavelength electromagnetic radiation used for therapeutic radiation.

Gene: a discrete DNA sequence that codes for a specific protein.

Genetic code: the complete gene sequence of an organism mapped out in its respective DNA code.

Genome: the total genetic content contained in a haploid set of chromosomes in single or multicelled organisms, in a single chromosome in bacteria, or in the DNA or RNA of viruses; an organism's genetic material.

Genomics: the study of genomic instability.

Her-2/neu: a gene found to be overexpressed or amplified in some breast cancer cells; evaluated routinely for both prognostic and therapeutic significance.

HercepTest: a rapid laboratory test for Her-2/neu activity.

Herceptin: the drug developed to interfere with the Her-2/neu gene/protein

Hereditary: inherited from one's parents and earlier generations.

Histologic grade: a system that attempts to quantify a pathologist's subjective interpretation of a cell's degree of differentiation.

Homogeneous (homogeneity): uniform; composed of the same element; in reference to a tumor cell population, it means that the cells are of the same clone, in contrast to a mixed-cell population that would exhibit heterogeneity or be heterogeneous.

Hormones: biologically active chemicals that are secreted by one organ and that then travel through the circulation, where they exert effort elsewhere.

Hormone therapy: the use of hormones, hormone analogues, and certain surgical techniques to treat disease (in this case breast cancer) either on their own or in combination with other hormones or in combination with other methods of treatment; because breast cancer may be dependent on estrogen to grow, hormonal (antiestrogen) therapy can be an effective means of alleviating symptoms and retarding the development of the disease.

Hyperplasia: an increase in the number of cells in an organ or tissue (see ductal hyperplasia).

Imaging: a radiology technique or method allowing a physician to see something that would not be visible to the unaided eye.

Immune system: the biological system that protects a person or animal from the effects of foreign materials such as bacteria, viruses, and other things that might make that person or animal sick.

Implant: (breast implant)—a type of breast reconstruction where a breast mound is recreated by the insertion of a saline filled balloon under the muscle of the chest wall.

Incisional biopsy: surgical removal of a piece of diseased tissue for submission for pathologic review.

Infiltrating ductal carcinoma: (see invasive ductal carcinoma).

Informed consent: permission to proceed given by a patient after being fully informed of the purposes and potential consequences of a medical procedure.

Intraductal carcinoma: another term for DCIS.

Invasive ductal carcinoma: the most advanced presentation of a mammary duct cell cancer where it no longer respects the duct wall as a boundary but invades or infiltrates surrounding tissues, blood, and lymphatic channels.

Invasive lobular cancer: as mentioned previously except regarding mammary lobule cells.

Ipsilateral: on the same side.

Lactation: the production of a mother's milk by mammary tissue.

Lobular carcinoma in situ: not believed to be a cancer but a defect that is associated with mammary cancer.

Lobule: that portion of the mammary glandular tissue that produces milk.

Localized: restricted to a well-defined area.

Local recurrence: a relapse of breast cancer in the conserved breast, chest wall, or axilla ipsilateral to previously treated breast cancer.

Lumpectomy: the surgical removal of a focal area of breast cancer.

Lymph (also lymphatic fluid): the clear fluid in which all of the cells in the body are constantly bathed; carries cells that help fight infection.

Lymphatic system: the tissue and organs that produce, store, and carry cells that fight infection; includes bone marrow, spleen, thymus, lymph nodes, and channels that carry lymph fluid.

Lymphedema: the swelling of the arm ipsilateral to the treated breast often associated with pain and infection.

Lymph nodes: the small glands that occur throughout the body and that filter the clear fluid known as lymph or lymphatic fluid; lymph nodes filter out bacteria and other toxins, as well as cancer cells.

Lymphoscintigraphy: a radiographic imaging technique used to map lymph flow within the breast.

Magnetic resonance: absorption of specific frequencies of radio and microwave radiation by atoms placed in a strong magnetic field.

Magnetic resonance imaging: the use of magnetic resonance with atoms in body tissues to produce distinct cross-sectional and even three-dimensional images of internal organs.

Malignancy: a growth or tumor composed of cancerous cells.

Malignant: cancerous; tending to become progressively worse and to result in death; having the invasive and metastatic (spreading) properties of cancer.

Mammary: the glandular tissue of the breast.

Mammogram: an x-ray of mammary tissue.

Mammotome: a tool used to facilitate stereotactic breast biopsies.

Margin: normally used to mean the surgical margin, which is the outer edge of the tissue removed during surgery; if the surgical margin shows no sign of cancer, then it is a negative margin.

Mastectomy: surgical removal of the breast.

Medical oncologist: an oncologist primarily trained in the use of medicines (rather than surgery) to treat cancer.

Menopause: the condition associated with the decline in estrogen production during a woman's middle age.

Mesoderm: the middle cellular layer of the developing embryo that gives rise to blood, muscle, and bone.

Meta-analysis: a statistical method that combines many related but not identical clinical trial outcomes to assess meaningful trends in patient treatment.

Metastasis (plural is **metastases**): a secondary tumor formed as a result of a cancer cell or cells from the primary tumor site (e.g., the breast) traveling through the blood circulation to a new site and then growing there.

Metastasize: spread of a malignant tumor to other parts of the body.

Metastatic: having the characteristics of a secondary cancer.

Metastatic therapy: the treatment of proven and measurable metastases.

Microarray testing: the study of genes and proteins likely to predict cancer risk.

Microcalcifications: small calcium deposits, nearly invisible without magnification, found within some areas of DCIS.

Micrometastasis: metastases that are too small to be measured by conventional testing.

Modified radical mastectomy: the surgical removal of the breast and axillary lymph nodes through a single incision.

Morbidity: unhealthy consequences and complications resulting from treatment.

Mutation: a defect in a DNA nucleoside base sequence that can lead to altered gene expression.

Neoadjuvant: the use of a different kind of therapy before the use of what is considered a more definitive therapy (e.g., the use of neoadjuvant chemotherapy before surgery for breast cancer); neoadjuvant is contrasted to adjuvant, which relates to the use of another therapy after the more definitive therapy.

Neoplasia: the growth of cells under conditions that would tend to prevent the development of normal tissue (e.g., a cancer).

Nuclear grade: a system that attempts to quantify a pathologist's subjective interpretation of a cell's nuclear abnormality.

Nucleoside bases: the four characters representing the chemical code for DNA.

Oncologist: a physician who specializes in the treatment of various types of cancer.

Oncology: the branch of medical science dealing with tumors.

Organ: a group of tissues that work in concert to carry out a specific set of functions (e.g., the heart or the lungs or the breast).

Palliative: designed to relieve a particular problem without necessarily solving it; for example, palliative therapy is given in order to relieve symptoms and improve quality of life but does not cure the patient.

Palpable: capable of being felt during a physical examination by an experienced physician; in the case of breast cancer, this normally refers to some form of abnormality of the breast that can be felt during an examination.

Partial mastectomy: see lumpectomy.

Partial response: a 50% or greater decline in parameters that are being used to measure anticancer activity; parameters include abnormalities found using physical exams and laboratory and radiologic studies (see complete response).

Pathologist: a physician who specializes in the examination of tissues and blood samples to help decide what diseases are present and therefore how they should be treated.

Perimenopausal: the years of estrogen production decline that precede menopause.

Placebo: a form of safe but nonactive treatment frequently used as a basis for comparison with pharmaceuticals in research studies.

Plasma: the viscous fluid of blood where the blood cells are suspended.

Platelet: a blood cell involved in blood clotting.

Ploidy: a term used to describe the number or sets of chromosomes in a cell (see diploid and aneuploid).

Positron emission tomography: a scan using a radioactive isotope that is taken up by tumor tissue showing that the tumor is functional.

Primary systemic: see neoadjuvant.

Progesterone: a specific steroid hormone in the family of progestins secreted by the corpus luteum of the ovary and by the placenta; it acts to prepare the uterus for implantation of the fertilized ovum, to maintain pregnancy, and to promote development of the mammary glands; many tumor cells contain progesterone receptors; used in the treatment of hot flashes; an example of a progestin is Megace.

Prognosis: the patient's potential clinical outlook based on the status and probable course of disease; chance of recovery.

Prognostic criteria: features of a cancer that fall outside traditional staging criteria but nonetheless are predictive of outcome.

Progression: continuing growth or regrowth of the cancer.

Prophylactic: preventative.

Protein: one of three major chemical classes found in living matter along with fats and carbohydrates. The machines of cells.

Proteinomics: the study of proteins resulting from genomic instability.

Protocol: a precise set of methods by which a research study is to be carried out.

PSA (prostate specific antigen): a chemical found in the normal prostate gland that may elevate in the blood when the gland undergoes cancer transformation.

Quality of life: an evaluation of health status relative to the patient's age, expectations, and physical and mental capabilities.

Radiant energy: see electromagnetic spectrum.

Radiation oncologist: a physician who has received special training regarding the treatment of cancers with different types of radiation.

Radiation therapy: the use of x-rays and other forms of radiation to destroy malignant cells and tissue.

Radical mastectomy: the surgical removal of the breast and axillary contents as well as the pectoralis and vasculature.

Radiotherapy: see radiation therapy.

Randomized: a feature of clinical trials whereby participants are assigned to different treatments to remove investigator bias.

Receptor: a docking site that interacts with a ligand (e.g., estrogen); receptors may be on the cell membrane or within the cell cytoplasm or nucleus; estrogen receptors are examples; all cells have multiple receptors.

Recurrence: the reappearance of disease; this can be manifested clinically as findings on the physical examination or as a laboratory recurrence or as an imaging finding.

Red blood cell: one of three blood cell classes along with white blood cells and platelets; responsible for oxygen transport throughout the body.

Regression: the real or apparent disappearance of some or all of the signs and symptoms of cancer; the period (temporary or permanent) during which a disease remains under control, without progressing; even complete remission does not necessarily indicate cure.

Remission: the measurable repression or shrinkage of a cancer—may be qualified as partial, complete, clinical, etc.

Resection: surgical removal.

Response: a decrease in disease that occurs because of treatment; divided into complete response (remission), partial response (remission), clinical response (by exam), radiologic response (by imaging), pathologic response (by microscopic review), etc.

Ribosome: the organelle within a cell's cytoplasm responsible for protein synthesis.

Risk: the chance or probability that a particular event will or will not happen.

Salvage: a procedure intended to "rescue" a patient after the failure of a prior treatment; for example, a salvage mastectomy would be the surgical removal of the breast after the failure of prior radiation therapy and lumpectomy to prevent a local reoccurrence.

Screening: evaluating populations of people to diagnose disease early.

Segmental mastectomy: see lumpectomy.

Selective estrogen receptor modulator: a drug that selectively inhibits estrogen receptors of a specific tissue(s) while allowing the normal interaction of the estrogen with estrogen receptors at other sites (see SERM).

Sensitivity: the probability that a diagnostic test can correctly identify the presence of a particular disease assuming the proper conduct of the test; specifically, the number of true positive results divided by the sum of the true positive results and the false negative results (see specificity).

Sentinel lymph node: that node that is first in line to receive lymph drainage from a particular anatomic location.

Sentinel node biopsy: the surgical removal of the sentinel node following its identification by lymphoscintigraphy or enhancement by injected visible dye.

SERM: a drug that selectively blocks one estrogen receptor but allows other receptors at specific sites to function normally with estrogen; Tamoxifen and Raloxifene are examples of a SERM—it blocks the estrogen receptor in the breast and uterine tissue but allows the estrogen receptor in bone tissue to be operative.

Side effect: a reaction to medication or treatment (most commonly used to mean an unnecessary or undesirable effect).

Simple mastectomy: surgical removal of the breast without disruption of the axillary fascia or underlying muscles of the chest wall.

Specificity: the probability that a diagnostic test can correctly identify the absence of a particular disease, assuming the proper conduct of the test; specifically, the number of true negative results divided by the sum of the true negative results and the false positive results; a method that detects 95% of true cancer cases is highly sensitive, but if it also falsely indicates that 40% of those who do not have cancer do have cancer, then its specificity is 60% (rather poor).

S-phase: see flow cytometry.

Squamous cell carcinoma: squamous epithelial cells that have undergone cancerous transformation.

Stage: a term used to define the size and physical extent of a cancer.

Staging: the process of determining extent of disease in a specific patient in light of all available information; it is used to help determine appropriate therapy.

Stereotactic breast biopsy: a technique using radiographic imaging to guide the biopsy of a nonpalpable lesion.

Support drugs: medications that have no inherent anticancer activity but improve the tolerance and safety of standard treatment.

Symptom: a feeling, sensation, or experience associated with or resulting from a physical or mental disorder and noticeable by the patient.

Systemic: throughout the whole body; affecting the entire body.

Systemic therapy: a therapy designed to be effective throughout the entire body.

Targeted therapy: therapies designed to target unique molecular structures.

Taxanes: a class of chemotherapy drugs that includes brand names Taxol (paclitaxel) and Taxotere.

Therapy: the treatment of disease or disability.

TNM staging system: a system for quantifying the extent of malignancy by numerically "grading" the size and extent of the primary tumor, the degree of involvement of lymph nodes and the presence or absence of distant spread (metastases).

TRAM: a reconstructive procedure that builds a breast mound from the transabdominal rectus muscle.

Treatment: administration of remedies to a patient for a disease.

Tumor: an excessive growth of cells caused by uncontrolled and disorderly cell replacement; an abnormal tissue growth that can be either benign or malignant (see benign and malignant).

Ultrasound: sound waves at a particular frequency (far beyond the hearing range) whose echoes bouncing off tissue can be used to image internal organs (e.g., a baby in the womb).

Wavelengths: see electromagnetic spectrum.

White blood cell count: one of three classes of blood cells along with red blood cells and platelets; responsible for immune surveillance.

Index

A

acquired mutations, 19, 31
adenocarcinoma, 13
adjuvant therapy, 22, 56, 74–76.
   See also chemotherapy
Adjuvantonline, 69–72
adrenal glands, 62
adriamycin, 67
advanced cancer, 15.
   See also invasive ductal carcinoma
   locally advanced, 88–89
   metastatic breast cancer, 89–90
adverse effects of treatments
   chemotherapy, 59–60
   posttreatment surveillance, 91
   SERM (selective estrogen receptor modulator), 63
age of patient
   breast changes with, 26–27
   breast/ovarian cancer syndrome, risk for, 30
   density of breast tissue, 26
   mammogram recommendations, 2
   menopause, 12, 27–28, 62–64
   premenopause, 12, 63
   risk factor assessment, 30, 70
   screening tests for cancer, 26
   treatment planning, 36
aggressive cells, 14
alcohol link to cancer, 85
alternative therapies, 82–84
amino acids, 18
analysis. *See* research
anatomy, breast, 10–12
aneuploid tests, 56
anthracycline antibiotics, 67
antibiotics, anthracycline, 67
antiestrogen therapy, 61, 67
appearance of cancer cells, 57
armpit, lumps in, 27
aromatase enzyme, 63–64
   inhibitors, 63, 67
aspiration, fine-needle, 32–33
assessing outcomes of therapy, language for, 68–72
assessment, risk
   for developing cancer, 29–31, 85
   Gail Model, 87

prognostic criteria, 56
staging and grading, 52–57
surgical options, 44–46
for uninvolved breast, 46
asymmetry of breasts, 26–27
atypical ductal hyperplasia, 14, 31
axilla, 27, 88
   axillary sampling, 38–41, 46

B

baseline mammograms, 2
benefits of clinical studies, 68
benign breasts diseases, 27
bilateral mastectomies, prophylactic, 46
biologic principles of cancer, 6–22
   breast structure and function, 10–12
   carcinogenesis, 12–16
   cell structure and function, 6–9
   genetics, 16–20
   invasion and metastases, 21–22
biopsies, 26, 32–34
birth control pills, 31
blood supply to breast, 10–11, 20–22. *See also*
   lymphatic system
bone marrow stem cells, 67
bone scans, 91
BRCA, 29–30
breast cancer. *See* cancer
breast-conservation surgery, 40
breast ducts, 10–15. *See also* DCIS; invasive ductal
   carcinoma
   ductal hyperplasia, 13–14
   mutated duct cells, 15
breast implants, 47–49
breast lobules, 10–11
   lobular carcinoma in situ, 15
   lobular hyperplasia, 31
breast lumps. *See* lumps
breast/ovarian cancer syndrome, 29–30, 61
breast reconstructive surgery, 47–49
breast removal. *See* mastectomies
breast symmetry, 26–27
breast tissue. *See* mammary tissue
breast ultrasound, 26–27

contaminated margins, 45
core biopsy, 32–34
counseling, genetic, 30
CT (computed tomography), 28
cure probability, 53
cycles, menstrual. *See* menstrual cycles
cytoplasm, 16–18
Cytoxan, Methotrexate, and Fluorouracil (CMF), 67

D

damage, cell, 19–20
data, presenting to patients, 68–72
data analysis. *See* standards of care
database for staging, 53
DCIS (ductal carcinoma in situ), 14, 20–22, 73.
   See also treatment
   detection of, 14–15
   margin-negative DCIS, 45
   microcalcifications found within, 27
   risk throughout the breast, 45
decision making. *See also* tests and screenings for
   cancer
   clinical trials. *See* clinical trials
   genetic testing, 30
   informed consent, 30, 53, 68
   invasive ductal carcinoma patients, 44–46
   presenting data to patients, 68–72
   risk assessment. *See* risk assessment
   shared decision making, 71
   staging and grading, 52–57
   surgery-related, 19, 32, 38–41, 44–46
   treatment. *See* treatment
defects, genetic, 12
deformity and cancer detection, 14–15, 26–27
density of breast tissue, 26–28
detection of cancer.
   See tests and screenings for cancer
diet for cancer prevention, 85
differentiation process, 8–9
dimpling, nipple, 27
diploid tests, 56
dirty margins of lumps, 34
discharge, nipple, 27
distortion of breasts and cancer detection, 14–15,
   26–27
DNA, 16–21, 58–61.
   See also genes and genetics; systemic treatment
   disrupting drugs, 58–59
   mutations, 14, 19, 29–32
"Dose Dense," 77–78
dose for optimal chemotherapy, 67
drugs. *See also* treatment
   preventative, 85–87
   support, 67
ductal carcinoma in situ. *See* DCIS
ducts, 10–15.
   See also DCIS; invasive ductal carcinoma

ductal hyperplasia, 13–14
   mutated duct cells, 15
dye injections for lymph node evaluations, 40–41

E

early detection, 24–25, 87
ectoderm, 8
efficacy of treatments, 66, 72
electromagnetic spectrum, 42–43
embryo, development of, 8
endoderm, 8–9
enzymes in estrogen, 63
epithelial cells, 12–13
ER (estrogen receptor) status, 56–57, 63–64
estrogen, 64
   age and level changes, 11–12, 26, 63–64
   alcohol effects on, 85
   antiestrogen therapy, 61, 67
   aromatase enzyme, 63
   breast development, 11–12
   ER (estrogen receptor) status, 56–57, 63–64
   exogenous, as risk factor, 31
   Her-2/neu, 36, 57, 64–65
   post-menopause production, 63–64
   replacement therapy, 61–63
   tumor sensitivity to, 36
ethnicity, as risk factor, 19
evaluation
   alternative therapies, 83–84
   biopsies, 29, 32–34
   lymph nodes, 36–38
   staging and grading, 52–57
   standards of care process, 66–68
   of therapy, language for, 68–72
Evista, 63, 85–87
exams and detection of cancer, 14–15, 27, 47–49
excisional biopsy, 33–34
exercise and cancer prevention, 85
exogenous estrogens, 31
expanders, 47–49
experimental strategies. *See also* clinical trials
   alternative therapies, 82–84
   preventative treatments, 85–87
   screening tests for cancer, 28–29
exponential growth of cancer cells, 35
external beam radiation therapy, 45
external patches as risk factor, 31

F

family of cancer patients, risk for, 19, 29–32
fat content of breasts, 12, 26
fibrocystic disease, 27, 46
fibrous tissue, 11–13, 26–28
finding cancer. *See* tests and screenings for cancer
fine-needle aspiration, 32

stereotactic breast biopsy, 32–34
sterilizing breasts of cancer, 42–43, 45
stress, hormonal and physical, 11–13, 16, 20
suffering vs. survival, 89–90
superiority of treatments, 66, 72
support drugs, 67
surgery
    axillary sampling, 40–41
    biopsies, 26, 32–34
    breast-conservation surgery, 40
    chemotherapy before, 88–89
    choices, factors affecting, 19, 32
    complete axillary node dissection, 38–40
    complications, postoperative, 39, 48
    genetic testing, impact on decisions, 32
    hospitalization stay, postoperative, 49
    options for, 19, 32, 38–41, 44–46
    postoperative care and recovery, 48–49
    postoperative treatment. *See* treatment
    reconstructive surgery, 47–49
    removal of breast (mastectomies), 38–40, 45–46
    removal of lumps, 32
    surgical margins, 44–45
surgical drains, 49
survival estimates, 68–72, 89–90
swelling of breasts, 26–27
symptoms of breast cancer, 26–27
systemic treatment, 40, 51–78. *See also* invasive
    ductal carcinoma
    chemotherapy, 58, 65–67, 88–89
    ductal carcinoma in situ. *See* DCIS
    hormonal therapy, 61–63
    language of clinical outcomes, 68–72
    locoregional therapy, 44–46, 74
    postoperative complications delays, 48
    staging and grading, 52–57
    standards of care, 66–68, 73–78
    targeted therapy, 60–61, 64–65

T

tamoxifen, 63, 85–87, 91
targeted therapy, 60–61, 64–65
taxanes, 67
tenderness from menstruation, 26–27
terminology of clinical outcomes, 68–72
tests and screenings for cancer, 24–34. *See also*
    evaluation
    biopsies, 26, 32–34
    clinical findings, 26–27
    early detection, 24–25
    estrogen receptor (ER) status, 56–57, 63–64
    experimental tests, 28–29
    fibrocystic disease, 46
    flow cytometry for S-phase, 56
    fluorescent in situ hybridization (FISH), 57
    genetic testing, 29–30
    Her-2/neu, 36, 57, 64–65

hereditary cancer, 19, 29–32
lumps, evaluation of, 32–34
mammograms, 2, 11, 14–15, 24–27, 91
physical exams, 14–15, 24–25, 27, 91
ploidy, 56
posttreatment surveillance, 91
radiographic findings, 27–29
removing tissue for testing, 32–34
self-exams, 14–15, 24–25, 27
specificity and sensitivity, 26
ultrasounds, 26
therapeutic radiation, 42–43
therapies. *See* treatment
tissue, mammary, 8–9, 11–13, 26–28. *See also* cell
    structure and function; mammograms
    density of breast tissue and age, 26
    removing for testing, 32–34
TNM staging system, 53–56
total body therapies. *See* systemic treatment
toxicity, limiting of chemotherapy, 67
TRAM reconstruction (transplanted rectus
    abdominal muscle), 48–49
treatment, 35–49, 66–68. *See also* surgery
    adjuvant, 22, 56, 74–76
    adverse effects. *See* adverse effects of treatments
    alternative, 82–84
    chemotherapy. *See* chemotherapy
    experimental preventative treatments, 85–87
    history of cancer management, 38–41
    hormonal therapy, 61–63
    language of clinical outcomes, 68–72
    locoregional therapy, 44–46, 74
    mastectomies, 38–40, 45–46
    metastatic therapy, 22, 56
    neoadjuvant therapy, 68, 88–89
    palliative therapy, 89–90
    posttreatment surveillance, 91
    preventative, 85–87
    primary systemic therapy, 68
    radiation therapy, 42–43, 45
    reconstructive surgery, 47–49
    staging and grading prior to, 52–57
    standards of care process, 66–68
    support drugs, 67
    systemic. *See* systemic treatment
    targeted therapy, 60–61, 64–65
trials, clinical
    informed consent for, 68
    language of clinical outcomes, 68–72
    preventative treatments, 86–87
    randomized, 77
tubes. *See* ducts
tumors and lumps, 21
    detection of cancer, 14–15, 25–27
    evaluation of the breast lump, 32–34
    lumpectomies, 32–34, 38–39, 40
    treatment planning, 36, 52–57

U

ultrasounds, 26–27
unconventional therapies, 82–84
undetectable cancer cells, destroying, 56
unilateral nipple dimpling or discharge, 27
uninvolved breast, risk assessment for, 46
USPSTF (U.S. Preventive Services Task Force),
 86–87

V

vascular invasion, 21
vessels, blood, 10–11, 20–22. *See also* lymphatic
 system
visible defects in breasts, 26–27
vital organs affected by cancer. *See* metastases

W

wavelengths, radiation, 42–43
web resources for patients, 69–71
white blood cells, 36

X

x-rays. *See* mammograms

Photo Credits for Background Images:

DNA Model © Photodisc/Getty Images shown on pages 2, 29, 52, 58, 86, 91, and 103.

Molecular Structure © Lawrence Lawry/Photodisc/Getty Images shown on pages 5, and 66.

Red Blood Cells © Chad Baker/Photodisc/Getty Images shown on pages 6, 37, 101, and 107.

Ripples in Calm Water © Photos.com shown on pages 23, 82, 96, and 108.

Woman Giving a Self Breast Exam © LiquidLibrary shown on pages 24, 36, 49, 88, and 95.

Assortment of Pills (#2) © Photos.com shown on pages 68, 74, 79, 85, 98, and 104.

The Chapter Openers are composed of all of the images listed above.